Policy, People, and the New Professional

D1244865

CARE & WELFARE

Care and welfare are changing rapidly in contemporary welfare states. The *Care & Welfare* series publishes studies on changing relationships between citizens and professionals, on care and welfare governance, on identity politics in the context of these welfare state transformations, and on ethical topics. It will inspire the international academic and political debate by developing and reflecting upon theories of (health) care and welfare through detailed national case studies and/or international comparisons. This series will offer new insights into the interdisciplinary theory of care and welfare and its practices.

SERIES EDITORS

Jan Willem Duyvendak, University of Amsterdam
Trudie Knijn, Utrecht University
Monique Kremer, Netherlands Scientific Council for Government Policy
(Wetenschappelijke Raad voor het Regeringsbeleid – WRR)
Margo Trappenburg, Utrecht University, Erasmus University Rotterdam

Policy, People, and the New Professional

De-professionalisation and Re-professionalisation in Care and Welfare

Jan Willem Duyvendak
Trudie Knijn
Monique Kremer
(eds.)

Amsterdam University Press

In memory of Eliot Freidson (1923-2005), whose work has been a great inspiration for this book.

This publication has been made possible with the financial support of the Dutch Ministry of Health, Welfare and Sport, the Netherlands Organisation for Scientific Research, Royal Netherlands Academy of Arts and Sciences, the Netherlands Institute of Care and Welfare/Department of Social Policy, Verwey-Jonker Institute, The Amsterdam School for Social Science Research/University of Amsterdam and the Department of Interdisciplinary Social Science/Utrecht University.

Cover illustration: © Sake Rijpkema/Hollandse Hoogte
May 2005: Ouder Kind Centrum (OKC), Amsterdam, the Netherlands. This centre is a collaboration of various partners, including accoucheuses, maternity care, Municipal Health Services, health centres, and child welfare organisations services. Boy being examined by a doctor, while his mother and sister watch.

Cover design: Sabine Mannel/NEON Design, Amsterdam
Lay-out: JAPES, Amsterdam

ISBN-13   978 90 5356 885 9
ISBN-10   90 5356 885 9
NUR   740

© Amsterdam University Press, Amsterdam 2006

Table of Contents

Policy, People, and the New Professional:

An Introduction

Jan Willem Duyvendak, Trudie Knijn and Monique Kremer

In the 1970s and 1980s, scholars were loudly criticising the power and intentions of social professionals. Three decades later, one hears a different voice, that of professionals whose power, expertise and knowledge are being undermined, which is causing serious problems. During an interview, Bourdieu (1998) said that the right hand of the state does not know what the left hand is doing. In other words, technicians, bureaucrats and policymakers have no clue about the work of those who actually implement public policy, such as teachers, policemen and social workers. As a consequence, the knowledge of what is really going on in society is not shared with decision makers, who in turn do not acknowledge the specific character of socio-professional work. They do not distinguish between the logic of the market and professional logic: 'How can we not see, for example, that the glorification of earnings, productivity, and competitiveness, or just plain profit, tends to undermine the very foundation of functions that depend on a certain professional disinterestedness often associated with militant devotion?' (Bourdieu 2002: 183-184).

Bourdieu and other analysts of social policy point out that the role of professionals has been changed – or reduced – as a consequence of the restructuring of welfare states by way of marketisation and accountability, the redefinition of citizens into consumers, and an accentuation of client participation. New modes of governance have intentionally limited the discretionary space of professionals. Marketisation and the focus on consumer-led services stress the voice of users or consumers at the expense of professionals. Since clients have now gained both voice (by means of legal appeals and by 'turning organisations upside down') and exit options (by giving clients vouchers or money to choose their preferred services), professionals have lost autonomy and authority. This makes it difficult to intervene in people's lives, even when clients may need support (Tonkens 2003). Additionally, the stress on accountability forces professionals to live up to managerial and bureaucratic standards. These new forms of governance have changed the motivation of professionals, their workload and the content of their job (Clarke & Newman 1997; Exworthy & Halford 1999). Rather than behaving like professionals they are led by a new kind of consciousness, 'a dispersed managerial consciousness', as Clarke and Newman put it.

The most striking evidence for the change in climate is the fact that a leading critic of professional power, Eliot Freidson, published in 2001 a book in defence of professionalism, *Professionalism: The Third Logic*. He describes two dominant logics that have now overruled the logic of professionalism: bureaucracy and consumerism. What worries Freidson is not so much the restriction of the knowledge monopoly of professionals, but the fact that professionals are no longer supposed to be the moral protectors of this knowledge. If they can no longer decide how and where this knowledge is to be put to use, professionalism itself is at stake. 'Professionals have a claim of license to balance the public good against the needs and demands of the immediate clients or employers. Transcendent values add moral substance to the technical content of disciplines... While they should have no right to be the proprietors of the knowledge and techniques of their disciplines, they are obliged to be their moral custodians'. This is how Freidson's book ends (2001: 222).

Knowledge, authority, morality, expertise and skills to deal with social problems: what exactly is lost when the professional logic is undermined? What is, more generally, the problem according to the critics cited above? It seems that they want to warn us that a process of de-professionalisation is underway; they worry that the professional logic is no longer respected because of the intrusion of both market and bureaucratic logic. In this book many authors take the same position, at least as a starting point. De-professionalisation is not their last word, however. On the contrary, in-depth empirical analysis shows that reverse processes are underway as well, as re-professionalisation might also be at stake. Interestingly, many authors claim that trends such as accountability (Body-Gendrot), contracting (Knijn & Selten) and evidence-based work (Hutschemaekers) may in fact have rather positive effects, or are at least ambivalent effects. Being accountable implies that you can participate in forms of deliberative professionalism: what do you do as a professional and why? Resulting in what? In several articles, the authors stress that though new logics may have perverse side effects, the very idea of a pure professional logic that can only be polluted by other logics is an overtly theoretical, essentialist and pessimistic argument. Duyvendak and Uitermark make a more general claim that practices and logics/ theories are not directly related anyway. Hence, changes in ideologies and predominant logics are never fully reflected in professional practices because ideological changes tend to bounce back since people in practice can stick to traditions, professionals can intentionally refuse to adapt to the new morals, and so on. Professionals are not only passive objects of change; they themselves play a role in defining professionalism.

As far as the processes of de-professionalisation are taking place, it may also have been necessary to limit the discretionary space of professionals – or at least of some professionals in some contexts. Therefore, this book deals with several types of social professionals, in several countries. This provides the opportunity to look at the conditions under which professional change can be harmful or useful, and for whom in what context. We have not selected cases from specific countries in order to compare them – rather, we demonstrate that comparable tendencies occur in several Western countries, where processes of re- and de-professionalisation occur in relation to marketisation and bureaucratisation.

Inspired by the concerns of scholars like Bourdieu, Clark and Newman, and Freidson, this book brings together three political and academic debates that are hardly ever dealt with in one go: professionalism, changing people and policy. Which policies are influential to processes of de-professionalisation and re-professionalisation? Is the comeback of (the debate on) professionalism linked to the increased political and public attention to social issues all over Europe? How do clients change the content of professionalism? And perhaps most importantly: what are the interesting alternatives to improve the balance between professionals, policy and clients? Are there, for instance, possibilities for a coalition between professionals and clients to fight policymakers that want to control professionals – to fight policies that cause professionals to not be accountable to clients but to bureaucrats and politicians (Trappenburg)? Are clients interested in these sorts of coalitions, or are they just turning their backs on professionals by using the exit option? Let's start with the policy side.

Policy

The first debate is about policy changes. The classic welfare state is a thing of the past. In that welfare state, allocation took place via two routes: bureaucracy, in which each client received the same treatment or benefits, and professionalism, in which professionals owned the knowledge and discretionary space to do what they thought was best for clients, patients and other vulnerable or dependent citizens. Today governments want to organise less and less themselves. The role of the state is at stake, torn between reducing its governing power in the implementation of services and keeping control ('steering, not rowing', as the British say). This role is becoming chiefly legislative, facilitative and sometimes supervisory. Through monitoring and accounting, governments try to keep professionals from crossing boundaries. The implementation of services is increasingly contracted out to the market or to private non-profit organisations. Political democratic control decreases, since accounting and monitoring is put in the hands of quasi-autonomous non-governmental organisations. This entails a significant shift in the public responsibility for the common good and in the democratic control of public services.

New concepts and trends have entered the policy arena. Besides contractualisation we now have to add accountability, managerialism, marketisation, privatisation, bureaucratisation, and user-led services. These concepts and trends have affected state policy towards social services, education and health care. Increasingly, welfare states stimulate competition and efficiency in public services via a 'marketisation' that has changed both the process and the culture of social and care services. Given the fact that services are paid out of taxes, transparency has become important – not only because managers and politicians demand it: citizens too urge for more accountability. Accountability is therefore crucial in this process that inevitably limits the autonomy of professionals. Since decision-makers still want to know what is going on at the level of implementation, accountability and marketisation have often gone along with re-bureaucratisation (Exworthy & Halford 1999).

The chapter by Knijn and Selten shows the effects of contractualisation in the Netherlands. Looking at different sectors they conclude that contractualisation has become a serious feature of social services, education, health care, youth care and police work. It is not clear yet whether this improves the quality of public services or clients' satisfaction with these services. What is clear is that contractualisation increases paperwork, because a regulated market demands more transparency and more accountability than hierarchically led organisations. In this context, professionals experience a reduction of both their discretionary power and the time they can spend on clients' needs. They also experience distrust from the side of politicians and managers. So far, they have not succeeded in finding an alliance with clients, patients or other groups of vulnerable citizens, which is a precondition for re-professionalisation on behalf of the clients.

It is not without reason that welfare states have had to change. Democratisation has led to demands for greater transparency; service malfunctioning and a lack of choice have inspired marketisation. The monopoly of professionals has been intentionally dismantled. Professionals themselves, especially in care and welfare, partly agree with the focus on accountability because they themselves feel they have to account for their interventions, since their work is paid by public money. But the question is whether there is a good balance between the need for accountability and space for professionals, the need for innovation, and marketisation. Trappenburg argues that the 'correction' has gone too far. She argues that an 'audit explosion' has taken place in the Dutch health care system, that has become a societal neurosis. This started with a call for patients' rights and institutionalising democracy, moved to the quest for high-quality care on the cheap, and has now reached a situation of hyper-control. So, societal neurosis starts with democratisation and then takes a turn for the worse as a result of new public management reform involving bureaucratic marketisation. The new legislation on health insurance very clearly shows this. Health insurers as well as patient organisations now have to monitor and control the performances of doctors. Patient organisations also have the difficult task of controlling insurers. In addition, five other boards and organisations will have to monitor the insurance companies. Trappenburg sees three ways out: real marketisation rather than bureaucratic marketisation, more trust in professionals and a reduction of monitoring, and a new bond between professionals and client organisations.

Accountability itself is not the problem, but the fact that it has become a societal neurosis. Does this also apply to the trend of evidence-based medicine or evidence-based social work, instruments that are increasingly used by policymakers to select specific treatments for specific social, individual and medical needs? If it works, treatment will be paid for; if there is no proof or if there are cheaper alternatives, professionals cannot offer it to their patients, clients or communities. Speaking in a general sense, it may be argued that many of the new developments can have quite positive effects on the position of professionals as long as we are not blind to the perverting side effects. The evidence-based mode of work originated in England and the United States, and has been in use for quite some time in health care. In introducing this kind of method, the scientification of welfare work has recently been proposed. Evidence-based social work is an intriguing combination of behaviourist, positivist and empirical science with policy research (Jordan 2000).

Opinions differ as to the applicability and desirability of this strategy, particularly in social work. Jordan observes that the notion of evidence-based social work uses measurable changes in behaviour or outcomes based on clear policy aims. In social work practice, this is extremely difficult. Policy aims are not always clear and measurable. How to measure the growing involvement in a neighbourhood? Besides, it is not always easy to ascribe behavioural changes to specific interventions. A behaviourist design is virtually impossible because other factors that can influence results cannot be excluded. Gradener and Spiers stress in their chapter what many social scientists have argued that society is a poor environment for controlled experiments, and in contrast to nursing or teaching, social work is 'work in context', as the social worker often has the task of creating his own context; to mobilise communities.

The question also remains as to whether evidence-based social work is not diametrically opposed to customised care. Professionals claim that each client, each patient is different. This requires constant adaptations in the work process itself. Other social scientists have expressed a great deal of appreciation for the strategy of evidence-based social work because transparency increases, and by applying approved techniques and instruments, social professionals can finally prove the worth of their work. What's more, the quality of professional work will improve (see, e. g., Scholte 2003).

In their chapter, Hutschemaekers and Tiemens rightly make a distinction between evidence-based work as an ideology and as a practice. Whereas the first oversees all of the problems mentioned above, the latter might be useful in a tailor-made approach. In a non-dogmatic, pragmatic way, evidence-based practices might help develop more effective interventions with respect to the positions of both professionals and patients.

As this book will show, the appreciation of new strategies not only depends on the way they are implemented but also on the specific (country) context. In France, as noted by Body-Gendrot, there is a lot to say in favour of more transparency and evidence-based accountability to reduce the disciplinary power of professionals, for instance, while in other countries such new strategies are misused and produce all kind of negative side effects. Moreover, whether these new developments 'fit' cannot and should not be answered by generalising, sweeping statements. There are enormous differences within and between (health) care and welfare, for instance with regard to accountability and contractualisation. Sometimes these are almost standard health care situations, whereas in other domains of welfare, professionals have never even heard about these new tendencies.

People

A second issue is the changing clientele of professionals. More than many other occupations, the daily tasks of social professionals are directly related to social change. Two of the most striking changes are the informed and well-voiced clients who are now gaining power as consumers, and increasing population diversity. Although more clients are well informed – proto-professionalisation, according to De Swaan et al. (1979) – the fact that social diversity and even inequality have increased implies that many citizens are poorly informed among whom, for instance, many members of ethnic minorities. In addition, governments label citizens as customers and consumers, and in doing so influence the behaviour of people requesting services. If citizens get the message that they have to become more personal responsible, they believe they need more know-how to be in a better position to articulate their demands and be more assertive about getting them (Van den Brink 2002). What's more, people are reinforced in the positions they can assume. In the first instance, this entails the role of the individual as consumer, who now has many more choices as a result of the marketing of care to such a large extent and welfare to a lesser one (Clarke & Newman 1997; Knijn 1999, 2000; Tonkens 2003). Second, people are also encouraged to get organised as citizens. In social movements, they make an effort to exert an influence on political decisions (Stüssgen 1997; Duyvendak & Nederland 2006; Nederland, Duyvendak & Brugman 2003; Nederland & Duyvendak 2004). Third, people are expected to exert their influence as clients. With increased frequency, and often backed by legal stipulations, they can exercise a voice in client organisations and participatory boards (client councils) of service organisations; in addition, they are stimulated to make use of their right to file a complaint.

Kremer and Tonkens show in their chapter that not only the old role of the client – the patient – but also the new roles of consumer and citizen are problematic regarding four issues: development of knowledge, trust, authority and the public good. Each issue is undermined when professional logic receives less space. They argue that a more suitable role for clients is that of co-producers or participants. This provides an alternative to Freidson's professional logic, market logic and bureaucratic logic. When clients and professionals become co-producers in care and welfare, one can then speak of a new logic, that of democratic professionalism in which clients have more of a voice and that both the knowledge of professionals and their role as guardians of the public good are taken seriously. This approach also repairs the wounds of trust in the relationship between client and professional.

Not all citizens take the role of client or consumer passively, nor are these roles the same for everyone. Well-educated people are often more willing and able to actively take the role of consumer, citizen or client. However, there is no way of knowing what the differences between them are, i.e., the citizen or client role that individuals play. What we do know is that society has become more diverse in terms of culture, ethnicity and nationality. Some of these differences are closely linked to forms of inequality. Colour and class divisions overlap, disempowering people of colour who might have different needs and wants regarding care and welfare. In a context in which professionals have to deal with increased diversity, new strategies develop to solve or contain the most complex problems, often geographically concentrated in certain neighbourhoods of big cities. Relatively new topics become preponderant (safety, crime, and ethnic bonding instead of multicultural bridging) for which professionals have to find new solutions.

Maarten Loopmans demonstrates that the Belgian case of Opsinjoren, a community project, successfully changes indifferent citizens into compassionate neighbourhood residents. He shows that policymakers and professionals are important in this creation of the new local citizen. At the same time, new differences come to the fore. Professionals, it is argued, have played an important role in the 'multicultural drama', and not always for the better. Since front-line workers allegedly had a cultural relativistic approach, this has not helped people from migrant backgrounds to adjust to – or integrate into – modern societies that demand –as the dominant discourse nowadays claims - speaking the local language and taking on modern values. The Norwegian anthropologist Wikan (2002) has argued that professionals have not made it clear enough what the values of Western societies are. Such a reproach to professionals is also visible in Dalrymple's (2001) analysis: social professionals – especially doctors – hardly confront their patients with the fact that they are responsible for their own lives. They in fact do little to intervene.

Marleen van der Haar's chapter opposes this position. Social workers indeed struggle with diversity, but they do depart from the five anchors that are very much based on a Western European individualised society – one of them being self-empowerment. Although social workers take into account the social context of the individual, they try to move their clients towards the direction of change in which self-reflection and self-empowerment are crucial. In that sense, a new kind of well-developed paternalism may on its way back.

Professionalism

By the early 20th century, the sociologist Emile Durkheim has expressed worries about professional ethics in relationship to civic morals. Between 1890 and 1912 he has given several lectures on the issue that many years later – in 1957 – have been published. Later on, also the sociologists Parsons (1968), Freidson (1986) and Abbott (1988) – have been concerned about the content, power and meaning of professionalism. Durkheim was pleading for professionalism as the moral pillar of a society that has lost its social cohesion because of European wars, migration and the domination of economic rationality. In this interpretation, morality is central where professionals have a different moral position in society than 'ordinary citizens' or the state technicians and bureaucrats. Durkheim (1957) argued that professionals working for the state serve the common good, which is why they should mediate between the state and its citizens by setting a moral example. As 'secondary groups' they could help improve social cohesion, based on peer groups in which they develop and share professional knowledge and ethics. Late twentieth-century sociologists, by contrast, instead of morality, put the accent on power and expertise as the crucial aspects of professionalism. In Parsons' functionalist approach, the client-professional relationship was characterised by a division of knowledge and expertise in which the professional had both and the client had little of either (Parsons 1968). For Parsons, professional power was necessary for successful treatment. Scholars like Freidson (1986) studied professional dominance and saw, just as many others did, that it was power at another's expense, while Abbott (1988) showed how a profession constructs itself in modern societies, often in response and in contrast to other professions.

More recently, Freidson (2001) has supplied some key criteria of a profession, distinguishing five characteristics that combine elements of Durkheimian morality, Parsons' expertise and knowledge, and Abott's notion of jurisdiction. This together creates a body of knowledge and skills that is officially recognised as based on abstract concepts and theories, and requiring the exercise of considerable discretion; an occupationally controlled division of labour; an occupationally controlled labour market requiring training credentials for entry and career mobility; an occupationally controlled training program associated with higher learning, providing opportunity for the development of new knowledge; and an institution-based secular calling or vocation.

Many of the professionals in this book are often not considered professionals. The classic approaches to professionalism seldom refer to professionals working in the care and welfare sectors, especially because they do not live up to the explicit criteria of professionalism. The ideal types of professionals are doctors – who are also dealt with in this book – and lawyers. Their knowledge can be clearly distinguished, and they have strong organisations as well as inclusion and exclusion rules. Social workers, home care workers and nurses have different positions on the professionalisation scale, which differs from country to country and are often called 'semi-professionals'. If we look at the Freidson's five criteria, it is professional organisation and an occupationally controlled division of labour in particular which are often lacking. The problem is also that the expertise and knowledge is not always acknowledged. Care and welfare professionals struggle with the lack of recognition. This is partly due to the fact that the tasks of these professionals are closely related to what can be labelled as a fourth logic, which implies a family logic based on kinship, reciprocity, normative claims and bonding. Consequently, this family logic of care is per definition arbitrary, and in contrast to the logic of the state and the market it is never indifferent, objective or impersonal, and is still over-determined by gender, implying that moral imperatives result in unpaid care work by female kin (Knijn 1999, 2000). If the distinction between professional and family logic in the fields of care and welfare is diffuse, this will come at the expense of the status and valuation of professional work. Authors like Schön (1983), and Celia Davies in this book, show that we can describe specific skills and knowledge in the social and care professions, even though they do not fit into the dominant categories of knowledge. To regard social workers and care workers as semi-professionals rather than as employees gives a new perspective to the development of this kind of work.

Since the 1970s, social professionals have struggled with the attack on their intentions and its effects. The issue of power and abuse has also emerged. What happened is that the assumption that clients and professionals were both aiming for a better world was dismantled. It was argued that professionals were following their own self-interests – they just wanted to maintain their professional status – or merely disciplining their clients. Their work was not beneficial to their clients; it was merely done to control society's deviants from which the professionals profited. Surprisingly, many professionals agreed with this criticism on their position in society.

Hard-core professionals take part in this too. Vogd in his chapter shows how the medical profession is under siege. Based on a study of German hospitals, he concludes that medical specialists are losing their grip on the quality of their work, losing contact with their patients, and experiencing a loss of discretionary power. Due to managerial reorganisations, cutbacks and new work processes, professional dissatisfaction is growing. According to the specialists, the main losers are the patients, who are often unaware of the backstage problems doctors are facing. Interestingly, Celia Davies shows the contrary: de-professionalisation of doctors is not the right way to frame the issue. Doctors are still 'Heroes of Healthcare', who co-operate intensely with management in an attempt to control treatment. The promise of better health puts doctors on a pedestal that obscures their uncertainty, their ambivalence, and also their power. Davies pleads for new vocabularies to better understand the construction of the hero identity of doctors.

Clearly, in this last part of the book, the debate is about professionalisation and de-professionalisation. Keeping many of these contributions in perspective, we would prudently propose that re-professionalisation is the dominant trend.

Gradener and Spiarts, for instance, argue that professionals have to regain their self-confidence by improving their professional knowledge and skills. They plead for re-professionalisation via the use of a combination of formal knowledge and practice-based evidence (Van der Laan 2003), as well as creating a knowledge alliance with stakeholders such as social scientists, managers, trainers, policymakers, and of course their clients.

Noordegraaf most clearly supports this re-professionalisation perspective. In his analysis of the role of managers dealing with professionals, he shows how their discretionary power has increased – often in interaction with policymakers – mainly at the expense of executive professionals. He does however note that this re-professionalisation of some social professionals (their managers) is not necessarily a zero-sum game. Some managerial styles may increase the professionalisation of all professionals in care and welfare. His general thesis that a re-professionalisation process is underway is partly corroborated by other articles in this book. We say partly because in some professions, in some countries, de-professionalisation is still the dominant trend. But this trend can be stopped almost everywhere. That is the positive conclusion of this book.

PART I

POLICY

The Rise of Contractualisation in Public Services[1]

Trudie Knijn and Peter Selten Netherlands

H11   P16

H41 L33

D73

J45

Contractual governance, a term introduced by Yeatman (1994), is gaining ground in the social services. The concept refers to a fundamental change in the governing of social services. Governance implies a new way of directing and controlling the provision of services; the well-known expression 'steering, not rowing' means that governments are withdrawing from the direct responsibility of providing services themselves or from directly subsidising on an input basis non-profit organisations that are responsible for providing such services:

> Complexity, dynamics and diversity has led to a shrinking external autonomy of the nation state combined with a shrinking internal dominance vis-à-vis social subsystems... Governing in modern society is predominantly a process of coordination and influencing social, political and administrative interactions, meaning that new forms of interactive management are necessary. Governing in an interactive perspective is directed at the balancing of social interests and creating the possibilities and limits of social actors and systems to organise themselves. (Kooiman & Van Vliet 1993: 64)

Governments have changed governing services by splitting up purchasers and providers, by output financing and by outsourcing services. Consequently, new ways of control are needed to guarantee that public means are used efficiently, effectively, and according to the policy objectives that are set by the administration. One way to guarantee this is through contractualisation. The assumption behind contractualisation is threefold: reducing bureaucracy, improving quality and efficiency, and increasing flexibility and diversity. Contracts replace former bureaucratic hierarchical systems of control in order to guarantee that the partners who get the responsibility of providing services of general interest will actually fulfil this responsibility – regardless of whether these are private, public, for profit or non-profit partners. This tendency takes a different shape depending on the welfare state, on very specific fabrics of service systems, relations between governments, and the degree of corporatism in the provision of services. Path dependency is important here, as well as the political assumptions of the successive administrations.

In this chapter we explore the theoretical assumptions as well as the consequences of this trend towards contractual governance by analysing several domains of public services as well as the role of and effects on professionals in the Netherlands.[2] What are the consequences on the way these domains function on behalf of common interests, what does it mean for their identification with the public targets, and to what extent does it influence their daily work practices?[3] We explore whether a balance between an efficient use of collective means and high-quality services can be reached via contracts. The question is whether contracting partners – be it between the government and voluntary, non-profit or for-profit organisations, or between social services and their clients – can replace former bureaucratic hierarchies, input financing and professional discretion. The implications for the balance between quality of services and cost efficiency also have to be considered.

Finally – and this is the aim of our contribution – we will elaborate on what this new governance means for professionals working in organisations that have a contract in which performance indicators register outputs and outcomes. Does this happen at the cost of the quality of the professional work and autonomy of professionals, or does it by contrast support professionalisation and the visibility of professional work?

Catching Many Birds with One Stone

Contractual governance has many fathers; the tendency towards contractualisation can be attributed to the need to cut back welfare expenses and to the political ideology of a small state. Still, it would be too simple to explain the tendency towards contractualisation in the domain of public services by pointing to the growing influence of a neo-liberal ideology alone. It is also a reaction to claims of patient and client movements for better services, of demanding a greater say and a better choice, as well as distrust of (semi-)state service providers and their professionals. The policymakers' recognition of the claims of service customers fits perfectly with the overall tendency in the 1980s and 1990s to promote self-help, shrink public services, and administer care and welfare more efficiently. Many authors (Clarke & Newman 1997; Knijn 1999; Exworthy & Halford 1999; Freidson 2001) signalled that the comments on the deteriorating, inefficient and expensive welfare state have gained ground since the 1980s, and cleared the way for the introduction of market-based principles in public provisions. Neo-liberalism by way of what Pierson calls 'programmatic retrenchment' (Pierson, 1994) found entry into the public sector. According to Pierson, retrenchment is governments' exercise in blame-avoidance rather than in credit claiming. Clarke and Newman (1997) and also Newman (2001) show that managerialism and new governance accompany the process of retrenchment, finding expression in a new rhetoric. Words like efficiency, consumer's choice, business-like behaviour, client-oriented attitude, and competition became part of the vocabulary of politicians from almost all of the parties, as well as civil servants and public-service managers. Managerialism did prove to be more than just rhetoric; in the name of competition and efficiency, the status of professionalism changed and the staffing and governing of professional care institutions changed profoundly:

> It is charged that professions have monopolies which they use primarily to advance their selfish economic interests while failing to insure benefit to consumers, that they are inefficient, their work unreliable and unnecessarily costly. Strip away their protective licenses and credentials, urge some, and let there be truly free competition. Open the market to all who wish to offer their services. Consumers will separate the wheat from the chaff in such a market so that the best services and products will emerge at the lowest cost. (Freidson 2001: 3)

In addition to economic comments on the public services, moral arguments arose that pointed to the paternalistic attitude of professionals towards their clients and to the increasing power of professionals in the public domain. By using terms like 'expertocracy' (Van Doorn & Schuyt 1978), 'bio-politics or the disciplinary power of professionals' (Foucault 1978) and 'disabling professions' (Illich 1977), social scientists and philosophers[4] set the tone for a decade-long debate about the power of professionals and their tendency to privilege their own interests above the common good, display elitist behaviour by using professional jargon, disrespect their clients, and deny their clients' knowledge and needs. These comments indeed hit professional specialists in the public domain – medical specialists, lawyers, and psychiatrists as well as teachers and social workers – in their Achilles heel. Their professional ethics and expertise was being contested in the name of the liberation and emancipation of clients.

The critique of the bureaucratic-professional system of the welfare state thus came from both sides, the right and the left. Whereas the socio-economic comments on the welfare state were firmly formulated by the (neo-)liberals, the socio-cultural comments have to be situated on the left wing of the political spectrum. The anti-psychiatric movement (in particular in the Netherlands and Italy), autonomous feminist healthcare centres, and students protesting against university professors, all are expressions of the declining trust in and respect for the way professionals serve public interests and, even more, professionalism itself.

Pleas for individual autonomy, community-based self-help, and clients' free choice and responsibility – that is, new-communitarianism and its belief in substitution to the lowest level of communities – mixed up with neo-liberalism and its market beliefs has been a historical irony since the 1980s. Together they led to a restructuring of the welfare state's public services by introducing market principles in these services[5] (Duyvendak 1999; Knijn 1999, 2000). Indeed, neo-liberal and communitarian assumptions about the position of the recipient, support-supplying mechanisms and how to meet demands differ fundamentally, but they share an aversion for the welfare state and its professionals. This was manifested in contractualisation, a new way of governance that organises state control on professional work through monitoring, auditing, performance indicators, evaluation and benchmarking (Clarke & Newman 1997).

Three Levels of Contractualisation

Contractualisation takes different shapes, and although we signal a general tendency, it remains crucial to distinguish three types of contracts: Between the government and providers of services that are in the general interest, between chain partners who co-operate in fulfilling a general interest, and between organisations that provide public goods and their individual clients.

Governments Contracting Service Organisations

National and local governments are increasingly outsourcing services to private companies and changing their relationship with non-profit organisations. This involves hardcore organisations such as public transport and electricity companies, as well as soft services of general interest such as the police, schools, hospitals and homes for refugees. Such services remain funded by collective means (with tax money). As governments remain responsible for their accessibility and quality, they bind organisations by contracts to deliver services of general interests. Governing at a distance by contract replaces the bureaucratic top-down hierarchy in which politicians are directly accountable for reaching policy targets. The expectation is that by contracting non-state organisations, expenses can be controlled, competition increased and services innovated, diversified and improved (Smith & Lipsky 1994).

Three side effects have to be mentioned. First one must beware of the risk of a democratic deficit, implying that the responsibility for public services falls between two stools. In a recent report on investing in government, Kohnstamm (2004) signals that politics is losing its grip on zelfstandige bestuursorganen (ZBOs/quangos: Quasi-Autonomous Non-governmental Organisations) that became independent providers of public services in fields such as immigration, refugee services, student grants and social security. Given the common interest of these services and because of citizens' rights to primary goods, the author explicitly pleads for the return of responsibilities to the political level – the government and its departments. The debate continues; some agree that governments are accountable for public services, others argue that we are facing an experiment that needs to fine-tune the contracts between governments and the quangos and other contracted partners.

A second side effect is that by splitting up purchasing and providing, state institutions lose their grip on the process of delivery. Nuis (2004) has pointed out this risk. The splitting up of purchasing and provision responsibilities frees ministers and civil servants from the accountability of the delivery process. However, Nuis found that courts and judges were too easily accepting evidence collected by private security organisations without checks and balances on the processes of evidence-collecting. Moreover, judges and the courts seldom check the private interests of those paying for the information. Citizenship rights as well as the constitutional state are at stake here. The process of delivering is also under discussion in the field of immigration policy. Democratic representatives feel that, although they agree on the immigration policy assumptions, the process of judging individual cases has been escaping from democratic control since it was outsourced to the quango, the Immigration and Naturalisation Service (IND). The national ombudsman has held the minister of immigration responsible for the IND's refusal to make juridical decisions in about 1100 individual cases.

Sennett (1998) puts the lack of responsibility for the delivery process in a wider perspective by stressing that current ways of governing, through both large corporations or state bureaucracies, are characterised by a neglect of the complicated process of implementation and performance. Though he may have too romantic an image of 'good old leadership', it cannot be denied that in the past governments took more responsibility for the process of reaching the targets they set. At present, policymakers are more focused on outcomes, leaving the complexities of implementation to the service providers.

The third side effect, as De Bruijn (2001), Gilbert (2002) and Dahrendorf (2004) note, is that contracts only have meaning if they are made operational by way of performance indicators. Contracts can have a perverse impact if they are either too detailed or too open. If they are too detailed they result in managerial bureaucracy, undermine professional discretion and neglect professional knowledge; if they are too open, the purchasing state is unable to control the relationship between price, quality, and outcomes of the services. There is also the risk of fixing indicators in such a way that they can always be reached. We will turn to this point later.

Given these comments, it remains uncertain whether programmatic retrenchment by way of outsourcing public services to commercial and non-profit organisations with contracts and leaving control of the implementation of social policy to such quangos will indeed result in more efficient, cheaper, customer-oriented and tailor-made services. Blame avoidance that results in a democratic deficit, and detailed performance indicators that result in managerial bureaucracy and in strict control on professional work do not exactly guarantee high-quality public services.

Contracts between Chain Partners

When the central direction of public services declines and substitution becomes a political target, local public and private partners have to cooperate to avoid fragmentation. Partnerships are developed among chain partners, for instance, in (health) care for the elderly between intramural, extramural and voluntary organisations (transmuralisation), among varied organisations that share a common interest, such as local housing corporations, social work and home care organisations that develop services together, or by way of multidisciplinary case management teams of social workers, youth workers, the police, and schoolteachers that offer guidance to pupils at risk.

Such networks and partnerships have grown in importance since the late 1980s. The intentions and motives often are to improve the quality of public services, to avoid fragmentation and overlap, to work more efficiently, and to stimulate innovation. Contracts can contribute to the cooperation of partners because they help clarify common targets, visibility and accountability of the joint efforts. However, they will have the opposite effect when they are too focused on outcomes and do not take into account the complicated process of attaining trust, becoming familiar with each other's work culture and adjusting work practices. In the context of a contract culture, there is the risk that each of the co-operating organisations prioritises its own targets above those of the partnership. Hence professionals participating in the partnership may be confronted with contradictory performance indicators. Therefore, according to Newman (2001), the contractualisation of partnerships demands accountability, in particular by creating proper structures and transparency, focusing on clear objectives, flexibility by adapting quickly to changing conditions, pragmatism in meeting targets and delivering visible results, and sustainability by fostering participation and building consensus. Newman signals that the different imperatives for partnerships are not necessarily reconcilable. Flexibility and pragmatism may obstruct accountability, and the need to reach short-term targets may frustrate the long-term process of sustainability.

Aside from these conditions, professional work in the context of the contractualisation of partnerships is rather complex if ultimate responsibilities remain fluid. Recent 'accidents' in the youth care sector in the Netherlands, where children were killed by their parents while about ten different youth care organisations were involved with the family, show again that blame avoidance is a great risk if no one has the ultimate responsibility. This is how the suggestion of introducing case managers evolved, implying another risk – that of creating a new class of professionals, the managing professional who instead of helping clients directly is mainly showing them their way through the diffuse labyrinth of chain partners.

Contracts between Public Service Organisations and Individual Clients

Former paternalistic or authoritarian relationships between doctors and patients, teachers and pupils, or social workers and clients no longer meet the demands of emancipated clients, nor are they a guarantee for efficient support for those clients who are unwilling to make good use of the services they need to become participating citizens. Hierarchical relationships between professionals and clients are increasingly substituted by formal contracts. These contracts are used in youth care, for instance, where delinquent boys are required to sign a contract that they promise to take part in re-socialising projects in exchange for less punishment. Secondary schools have introduced so-called pest-contracten (harassment contracts) to reduce harassment. Of course, interventions on behalf of clients, pupils, or patients can only reach their objectives if these subjects are motivated to follow the rules of the game and participate in lessons and treatments that do not always appear to be in 'their best interest'. Since public services cannot permit too many dropouts, do not have time or fail to persuade clients, and have to account for their results in terms of 'production', they can either refuse treatment to demotivated persons or bind them to contracts. Both strategies are applied. Hence, many youngsters left school (64,000 in the Netherlands in 2004) without having any other options while psychiatric patients with numerous problems are left in the middle. In these cases, contracts seem to offer a better perspective though their meaning is mainly symbolic. Problematic pupils, welfare clients, psychiatric patients and drug addicts are often impressed by the signing of a formal document in which their rights and obligations are detailed, and will be more aware of the goals and implications of the project they are participating in. Nevertheless, effectuation of the contracts remains difficult and sanctions often consist only of exclusion. It is problematic that these contracts suggest equality between the supplier and user of services even though they are mostly one-sided; given the circumstances, the user is basically compelled to sign the contract and sanctions for a service organisation that does not fulfil its part of the agreement are seldom included. In addition, professionals often consider the contract as either inadequate or too rigid. The contracts are mostly framed by a specific category of professionals, the indicators, who are not the ones involved in providing the service. Since social work, youth care, and therapy are interactive processes, professionals working with clients experience a dilemma when their expertise tells them to deviate from the original contract. Should they stick to the formal contract or quietly do what they think is appropriate in that specific case?

Contractualisation, Performance Indicators and Professionalism

Contractualisation implies a shift in trust. It expresses that professionals in the public sector can no longer be trusted simply because of their training, expertise and professional ethics. These 'street level bureaucrats' (Lipsky 1980) will have to prove loyalty to the public good as well as the effective and efficient delivery of services. The trust in providers of services is in need of a new foundation. Newman (2001) has noted a shift from a society in which trust was based on (status-based) identity towards a society that is characterised as a calculus-based trust. Tonkens (2003), as well as the Dutch Advisory Council on Government Policy (Wetenschappelijke Raad voor het Regeringsbeleid/WRR, 2004), have even spoken of an 'organised distrust' of social work professionals. An identity-trust-based society assumes that those organisations and professionals who have a task in the delivery of public services identify with the common interest to such an extent that they do their very best to devote themselves to realise their public tasks and obligations. Shame and scandal because someone has neglected one's public duty are the sanctions. Professional honour and ethics at one time worked as positive stimuli to fulfil one's task properly. Social controls by the public and fellow professionals were considered to be enough to maintain professional ethics and commitment to the public good. A calculus-based trust assumes that honour, shame and scandal have become less important. Professionals, like all other human beings, are motivated mainly by economics-based rational motives and can only be compelled to fulfil their responsibilities by way of the old stick-and-carrot method. This means that it is wise to draw up a contract in which all of the tasks, goods, and services are described, calculated, and settled.

What are the implications for professionals of vertical contractualisation between the government and services on behalf of the common interest, and between service organisations and clients on the one hand, and horizontal contractualisation between partners co-operating on behalf of the general interest on the other? We have already observed that contractualisation is founded on the premise of calculus-based trust, assuming that professionals are only motivated by rational motives and can only be compelled to fulfil their responsibilities through a fear-and-reward mechanism. Although performance contracts are formally drawn up between organisations or between organisations and their clients – not between the government and individual professionals – they have repercussions on the relationship between the management of organisations and the professionals working in these organisations.

Given that the organisation has to meet the requirements of the contract, it will also have to deliver an overview of its 'products'. Reporting on one's performances, results and outcomes implies collecting indicators from the organisation's employees, so that professional workers will be confronted with performance indicators and this will result in managerial bureaucratisation. Performance contracts often contain detailed agreements about the services ('products') to be delivered. These agreements also include figures of the number of clients, a detailed description of treatments, price or costs, and the time needed to provide such services or treatments. A covenant between the Home Secretary and the Police District of Zuid-Holland-Zuid, for instance, has demanded an increase of 1000 reports over four years. The Dutch Federation of Hospitals has contractually agreed to a 2.3% increase in 'production' between 2004 and 2007 (Groei door doelmatigheid [Growth by Efficiency] 2004). Client managers (Personal Advisers) at social offices have to deliver an x-number of welfare recipients to the contracted for-profit employment integration company per week, and, in the future, general practitioners will have to present the DBCs (Diagnose Behandel Combinatie/Diagnosis-Treatment Combination) for each individual treatment to insurance companies (see also Vogd in this volume regarding Germany).

The principle of the registration of results, performance and outcomes is becoming a daily practice in many public service organisations. In addition to the employment contract, professionals often have supplementary agreements on the exact 'products' the individual employee needs to deliver. Home care workers, guardians, client managers, university teachers, general practitioners and psychotherapists also have a caseload or a standard number of clients they have to help within a fixed span of time. Police officers and academic researchers have to meet 'targets', such as certain number of tickets issued annually or articles published in refereed journals. Their functioning is evaluated based on measurable output. For managers as well as clients, and maybe even for professionals themselves, this has the advantage of transparency; all participants know what to expect. It also creates equality among professionals; the standard is well known and often clearly communicated within an organisation, and professionals have to perform according to these standards. Two comments can be made here. First, since these professionals work with people who do not always fit the standards – in particular those who need special attention – they often experience increases in work pressure. Second, due to managerial bureaucratisation, professionals often complain about how much more time they spend on paperwork at the expense of the time they can spend on their clients. Performance contracts not only set standards for outcomes, they also concentrate on the process and procedures of delivering products:

> Demands have also increased for programmatic accountability. As a condition of maintaining funding, public agencies and other sponsors insist that contract agencies develop and keep track of indicators of program success. (Smith & Lipsky 1994: 81)

The aforementioned police contract thus contains detailed agreements on better accessibility of police stations (in person and by phone). Hospitals and home care organisations guarantee a reduction of waiting lists, universities promise a minimum of contact hours between teachers and students, and child welfare organisations have developed protocols on the steps that have to be taken from admission to diagnosis and therapy. At the level of the professional, this means that procedures are standardised and appointments and results have to be recorded meticulously. This produces no end of figures and other data that are not only used as the accumulated results of the organisation as a whole, but can also show the average performance per capita.

The question is what influence such procedures have on the work ethic of the individual professional. A rehabilitation employee said that the transition from input to output financing was the most important change in working conditions during the last years:

> Today we speak of delivering products instead of helping people... The introduction of the CVS (a computerised protocol in which all appointments and data about one particular client are registered) has brought about a more uniform way of working. You have to follow all the steps in the system and there is less freedom to make your own decisions.

This on-going standardisation of processes and procedures has a disciplining effect on the work of professionals. Whether it reduces their discretionary space remains to be seen. A police administrator and a school policymaker both note that there is still enough room for individual decision-making within the framework contradict the view of the rehabilitation employee. Despite strict procedures there were also large differences between probation officers regarding decisions that concern when and how to formally end supervision when clients failed to comply with the agreements.

The proponents suggest that contractual relations between organisations result in better products as well as more, quicker and cheaper output. In almost all sectors of social work and public services, performance indicators contain detailed prescriptions on how to act in given situations. Hence these performance instruments contain regulations on the professional work itself as well as quantitative prescriptions concerning managerial tools for the delivery of services, such as the caseload or accessibility. The Child Protection Agencies have developed the BARO (Basis Raadsonderzoek in Strafzaken/Basic Court Research in Penalty Cases), a standard questionnaire that has to be used by all staff members to make a diagnosis and to create a database for future treatments. This instrument was explicitly introduced to prohibit interpretation differences between staff members. Risk-taxation instruments are prescribed in mental hospitals where criminals are treated. Several measuring instruments and protocols according to which patients have to be examined are being developed for the medical profession in particular. This includes the DBCs (Diagnose Behandel Combinatie/Diagnosis-Treatment Combination) and the Basisset Prestatie Indicatoren Ziekenhuizen (Basic Inventory of Performance Targets for Hospitals). The development and use of such qualitative performance indicators is often part of the performance contracts organisations have with the government.

It is clear that these detailed prescriptions of how to deal with clients' questions and problems do impose restraints on the autonomy of professionals. They not only have to comply with standard procedures, there is also interference with their professional habits. Some professionals, like psychiatrists, consider the regulation of having to indicate the specific diagnostic instruments they have chosen as a violation of their professional and even personal integrity. This does not mean that they are not willing to discuss these methods with colleagues, but they resist prescription. On the other hand, this development is also outlined as an improvement of the conditions of employment of professionals and even as a way of reinforcing their professional standards. Two lines of argument are being followed here. One argues that a detailed procedure or protocol can be very helpful in providing a diagnosis or deciding on the proper care. Alternatively, a standardised procedure is defended with the argument that it protects the professional against unjust allegations. After all, the records can now show when and by whom a mistake was made, and who is responsible. We should therefore be careful with the claim that performance targets simply undermine the professional's autonomy.

Interestingly, performance contracts not only take into account the product and the way it is made, but also its reception among clients. Market economy concepts and procedures have even found their way into the area of client satisfaction, which has become an important indicator of a service organisation's quality. For this reason, almost all performance contracts include commitments to measure the client's opinion (nowadays defined as 'consumer') on the services delivered. The aforementioned Police Covenant, for instance, literally stipulates that 'in 2006 the percentage of inhabitants that is "very content" with their contact with the police has be substantially higher than in 2003 (67%)'. Public service organisations are nowadays dealing with external audits that include client satisfaction. This focuses managers on staff performance. The (quasi-) contractualisation of the relationship between organisations and consumers changes the relationship between professionals and patients/clients. When clients are continuously approached as if they are autonomous consumers in the care market, one should not be surprised if they begin considering the professional as a mere market vendor.

Transparency, Performance Indicators and Professional Discretion

Obviously, performance indicators play a crucial role in the improvement of responsibility and accountability in public services (De Bruijn 2001). They improve the transparency of service organisations as well as of the individual professionals working in these organisations. Organisations can also make use of performance indicators to start a process of continuous learning. Performance indicators can contribute the overall valuation of the quality of the organisation, its work processes and the quality of the employees, and can subsequently be used to reward or penalise good or poor performance. Among the organisations co-operating in partnerships, these indicators can form an additional basis for a process of comparing tasks, activities and results (benchmarking), and selecting 'best values'. Finally, performance indicators can contribute to a client's informed free choice. If parents receive information about average school results, this can guide them in the selection of a school for their children; when patients have transparent information about the quality of hospitals, they can make an informed choice of where to go for treatment.

Performance indicators may also have an adverse or even perverse effect, as De Bruijn (2001) argues. This goes for performance indicators measuring results as well as for those that measure processes. Measuring and rewarding output can encourage strategic behaviour, such as letting as many students as possible pass their exams or refusing clients with a low expectancy of treatment success. It can also slow down innovation and discourage professional habits, because the exploration of new subjects and methods takes time and does not produce immediate results. This danger also exists if only the procedures are measured, for instance, when a peer review is required as part of any course of action. According to De Bruijn, professionals are mutually dependent and therefore inclined to argue in favour of the familiar. Avoiding professional resistance demands combining output and process measurement as well as professional involvement in the construction of the performance indicators and in carrying out the evaluation process.

Gilbert (2002) on the one hand, makes it clear that performance indicators will have to be very detailed to reach the maximum transparency that the government and consumers expect. If the components of services offered and the quality of the products are not tightly framed and not well-described, providers will demand the highest price for a diminished quality of service (still under the condition of calculus-based trust). On the other hand,

> [i]f the administrators are able to break down each component into its smallest segment, rationalizing services and leaving providers less room to manoeuvre... They also leave less room for professional discretion. Under this

system, social care that heretofore involved in a holistic process informed by professional values and expertise is transformed into a series of discrete procedures bridled by pressures to contain costs... (Gilbert 2002: 122)

How, then, does one improve the transparency of public services while still respecting professional knowledge, skills and discretion? One condition for this – and Hutschemaekers (2001) stresses that it is a crucial one – is that professionals envision directives, guidelines, and protocols that include performance indicators as part of their tools and instruments. Professionals own these instruments, and they should only use them to improve the quality of their work, for instance by using evaluations and scores in inter-professional discussions on how and why tasks are performed and how to improve their quality. This condition is, however, hard for all of the professions to fulfil, and contrasts with the goal of reaching the highest quality for the lowest price, which is an explicit aim of contractualisation. Our limited empirical evidence suggests differences between interlocutors. Members of the managerial staff envision indicators as managerial instruments more than as instruments to empower professionals and improve professional quality, so they tend to be more enthusiastic than members of the professional staff about this process. We also have the impression that higher-educated professionals such as medical doctors and university teachers are better equipped to influence the content of the performance indicators than semi-professionals such as police agents, elementary school teachers and child welfare workers are.

Another condition formulated by De Bruin (2001), based on the way some companies in the United States use the instrument, is that a 'culture of fear' should be avoided when implementing performance indicators. As long as fairness, justice, and protection are incorporated into the relationship between managers and professionals, performance indicators can result in an active evaluation of the work processes. The evaluation processes should not only include the work of the professionals but also commit managers to obligations and responsibilities. Reciprocity and trust are crucial aspects of the process.

Conclusion

Back in 1994, Smith and Lipsky (1994: 110-111) wrote:

Over time, contracting may reward agencies that offer low costs when quality of service remain difficult to judge. European countries with extensive government funding of nonprofit agencies, ... such as Holland and Germany, do not really have a contracting system. Instead, nonprofit agencies have almost monopoly status within their service jurisdiction... As a result, agencies in these countries do not experience the bidding and contract competition character of the United States, which places downward pressure on agency costs and creates incentives for deprofessionalization.

In this chapter, we have shown that times have changed; contractualisation has become a serious feature of the relationship between managers and professionals and between governments and non-profit organisations in the Netherlands as well. The tendency can be found in education, social work, health care, youth care, home care and police work. We have stated that this tendency has many fathers and we have explored some of its merits and concerns. Blame avoidance by programmatic retrenchment is not only a cause but can also be the result of contractualisation if the ultimate responsibilities of the contractual partners are not strictly defined. This risk is already visible in the democratic deficit of the quangos and in the malfunctioning of chain partners, for instance in youth care, so an option would be to develop better contracts when a hierarchical bureaucracy is set aside. On the other hand, contractualisation obviously has consequences for the character of professional work: Transparency as well as perversity may increase, and excessively strict performance indicators damage professional discretion and increase paperwork, undermining professional standards for good services. Caught between the demands of client movements' for free choice and a greater say on the one hand and governmental demand for reduced expenditures, professionals in public services face a prisoner's dilemma – an exit option is not available. Raising their voice through self-confident reprofessionalisation may help reclaim professional discretion on behalf of those clients who need their support.

Notes

1   We are grateful for Giel Hutschemaekers comments on the first draft of this paper.
2   Although we realise that most social services employees are semi-professionals, according to the Freidson (2001) and Hutschemaekers (2001) standards for professionalism, for the sake of simplicity, we will categorise them as professionals and pay attention to the vertical hierarchy of professionalism at the end of this article.
3   The chapter is based on theoretical and empirical material that we collected during several years in which we taught a course on 'Social policies and care arrangements' within a program of the Interdisciplinary Social Science Department of Utrecht University. Students participating in this course submitted papers on the working of contractualisation in several social areas and public services in which they describe the mechanisms of contractualisation, such as the introduction of performance indicators and the way organisations and their professionals deal with new governance. For the empirical part of the chapter, we have selected some of these student papers,

realising that they only represent a small selection of the experiences regarding the issue at stake:

Bartray, Annemarie, 'Kwaliteitszorg in het hoger onderwijs'.

Bolscher, Marieke, 'De professional binnen de raad voor de Kinderbescherming'.

Burg, Jessica van der, 'BPO en verschillende logica's'.

Jansen, Floor, 'Van helder naar transparant. Een onderzoek naar de effecten van beleidsverandering bij de reclassering in Groningen'.

Ketelaar, Nicole, 'Protocollen: controlemiddel of aantasting van de discretionaire ruimte van de professional?'

Konings, Tonnie, 'UWV Gak: Aanbesteding in reïntegratie'.

Prickaerts, Judith, 'Interventies voor ernstig delinquente jongeren'.

Renema, Lida, 'Vastleggen of vrijlaten? Een case-study naar de implementatie van vraaggericht werken en accountabality in de jeugdhulpverlening'.

Sijl, Liselore, 'Verzakelijking in de welzijnssector'.

Terpstra, Oscar, 'Politie en prestatie'.

4   In the Netherlands, the philosopher Hans Achterhuis (1979) played an important role in this debate; his book *The market of welfare and happiness* accused social workers of creating illusions about what social work could do for individuals and communities in order to keep their business going. According to him, clients ended up even unhappier than before they were 'supported' by social workers. This book undermined the self-confidence of a whole generation of social workers in the Netherlands.

5   For contractualisation of gender relations, see Gerhard, Knijn and Lewis (2002).

Evidence-Based Policy

From Answer to Question

Giel Hutschemaekers and Bea Tiemens

I 11
I 18

Netterlands

Between the years 1980-1990, the Osheroff case aroused the emotions of many psychiatrists (Kaasenbrood 1995: 10-15). Osheroff suffered from serious depression. Following the failure of treatment with medication, he was admitted to Chestnut Lodge,[1] where he was treated for seven months using clinical psychotherapy without medication. His condition deteriorated to such an extent that his family requested a different treatment. When this request was not honoured, the family decided to have Osheroff transferred to another clinic. Here he was treated with medication. Osheroff's condition quickly improved, and after three months he was discharged completely free of symptoms. However, this is the beginning and not the end of the story.

Osheroff thought he had suffered injuries while at Chestnut Lodge and decided to take them to court. The absence of efficacy studies on psychotherapeutic treatment should have been reason enough for Chestnut Lodge to treat him with antidepressants. The effecacy of these drugs is firmly established (Klerman 1990). The counsel for the Chestnut Lodge defence argued that the claims of the efficacy of medication was too limited. Clinical treatment should also be aimed at professional standards and the 'collective sense of the profession' (Stone 1990).

The Osheroff case illustrates in a nutshell the main aspects of the later controversy on evidence-based policy. Evidence-based policy takes the view that professional practice should be in concordance with scientific evidence. This policy is widely accepted to the extent that it has reached the characteristics of a paradigm. However, it is not clear what this paradigm actually looks like (Sehon & Stanley 2003). Do we all consider the same paradigm when we talk about evidence-based policy? Definitely not. In this chapter we will describe two different, basically opposite, views on evidence-based policy: one starts with the answers and the other with the questions.

First Impressions of Evidence-Based Policy

The term evidence-based has become a familiar one over the last 15 years or so. While in 1992, the reputed databank Medline contained only one article on the subject, this number had risen to over 13,000 by February

2004 (Strauss et al. 2005). In addition to evidence-based medicine, many other variants on the term have been introduced in recent years. Professionals in mental health care refer to 'evidence-based mental health' and the nurses to 'evidence-based nursing' (Cox et al. 2004).

One characteristic of this evidence-based approach is the viewpoint that care should be based on scientific research results (Offringa et al. 2000). An intervention is evidence-based if scientific research has proved the intervention to be 'effective', and if as far as it is known there is no alternative therapy that could lead to the same result. Scientific research results are superior to the experiences found in daily practice. This is true because statements on illness and health that derive from strict and monitored conditions are far more solid than the judgements of professionals, which are unintentionally but too often based on opinions (Kaasenbrood 1995). In this respect, 'evidence-based' is preferable to 'practice-based', 'experience-based', or 'opinion-based'. These alternative working methods are based too much on coincidental traditions and habits.

In general health care, evidence-based medicine is generally accepted as a tool for professionals in order to provide better care (Haines & Donald 1996). In mental health care the reactions are mixed. In addition to unconditional support (Stout & Hayes 2005) there is also careful criticism (Kaasenbrood et al. 2004; Mykhalovskiy & Weir 2004). Professionals often treat the paradigm as a straitjacket, claiming that independent decision-making is the core business of professionals and that any decisions those professionals make depend on much more than scientific knowledge alone.

The loudest criticism comes from the social work disciplines (Bruce & Sanderson 2005; Gambrill 2005). According to Van der Laan (2003), evidence-based working implies that the professional competence is neutralised by rational operational management and is reduced to forms of pre-structured working methods. Evidence-based policy leads to professionals being turned into robot-like implementers of diagnostic instruments and interventions.

In the following sections we shall show that the controversies are related to the two different meanings evidence-based policy has for professionals in the health care sector (Sehon & Stanley 2003). First, we present the policy of evidence-based practice that strictly adheres to protocols and guidelines derived from science (the guideline approach). This is the policy to which most of the above-mentioned criticism is directed. Our case study analyses the new Dutch standards for good clinical care for those with anxiety disorders. The second policy is based on a method that enables professionals to work according to the latest scientific insights, independently weighing these insights in combination with their own expertise. We have called this the heuristic approach.

The Guideline Approach

In the guideline approach, evidence-based policy is seen as providing care in accordance with guidelines based on existing scientific knowledge (Timmerans & Kolker 2004). Guidelines are documents containing recommendations published by professional organisations that can support professionals (and nowadays also clients) in decision-making on the correct form of treatment (Eddy 1990). Up until the 1990s, these standards were mainly the result of intensive discussion between experts in the field concerned, and later became known as consensus-based (Kaasenbrood 1995). Although these standards do contain the state of affairs regarding knowledge, when used they often turned out to be the product of compromises that were made from behind a desk, and therefore hardly applicable in daily practice. The main feature that was lacking was the criteria to determine who was right. This meant that on a regular basis, the most tenacious and persevering expert would be able to push his opinion through into the standards.

In the late 1990s, new standards in the US, UK, and Australia became evidence-based, meaning that they were constructed on the basis of the levels of evidence (Hutschemaekers 2003). The levels of evidence were constructed by the Cochrane Association in the 1980s, and based on the authoritative book of Archie Cochrane *Effectiveness and Efficiency* (1972). Stated simply, these levels indicate the extent to which the effectiveness of an intervention is empirically grounded. Figure 1 shows the five levels of evidence that are currently distinguished:

Level of evidence

1a	Systematic review with homogeneity of RCTs
1b	Individual RCT with narrow confidence interval
1c	All or none*
2a	Systematic review (with homogeneity) of cohort studies
2b	Individual cohort study (including low-quality RCT)
3a	Systematic review (with homogeneity) of case-control study
3b	Individual case control study
4	Case series (and poor-quality cohort and case-control studies)
5	Expert opinion without explicit critical appraisal, or based on physiology, bench research or 'first principles'

* An all-or-none criterion is met when all of the patients die before the treatment becomes available, but some now survive with available treatement; or when some patients die before the treatment becomes available, but now none of them die with treatment.

Fig. 1 The levels of evidence (from Strauss et al. 2005: 169)

At the top of the hierarchical list of scientific knowledge are the outcomes from research according to the method of randomised clinical trials (RCT). A systematic review with homogeneity means that this review is free of worrisome variations in the directions and degrees of results between individual studies. The conclusion of such a review is therefore unequivocal. Characteristic of the RCT is its controlled and experimental nature. The effectiveness of a new intervention (experimental condition) is determined by comparison with an existing intervention or a placebo (control condition). Test subjects are randomly allocated to one of the two (or more) conditions. The intention of randomisation is to include patients in each condition who's characteristics can only differ by chance, because bias by patient or clinician selection has been ruled out. When this procedure is successful, outcome differences between patient groups can be assigned to differences between the treatment conditions.

In all of the following levels, there is less control in the design than the design of a RCT. The stricter the design and the smaller the chances of disturbing factors lead to harder evidence and a higher place on the ladder of evidence. Reliability and replication are more important according to this hierarchy than validity and representativity of the research results.

An Example: The Dutch Multidisciplinary Guideline for Anxiety Disorders

The Dutch multidisciplinary guideline for the diagnosis and treatment of anxiety disorders has been drawn up by experts from all the relevant professional organisations in mental health care: general practitioners, psychiatrists, psychotherapists, psychologists, nurses, social workers, creative therapists and psychomotor therapists (LSR 2003). Clients also participated in the creation of this guideline. All of the participating professional organisations as well as all of the participating client organisations have approved this guideline. The most important conclusions are summarised in flow charts. Here we present the chart for the treatment of obsessive-compulsive disorders (fig. 2).

When there is no comorbid depression, client and therapist can choose between two preferred treatment options: psychological treatment (i.e., exposure with response prevention) or pharmacological treatment (SSRI). Should the selected treatment not produce sufficient effects within the suggested period, then a different option is recommended. Should the effects of the treatment remain inferior, then a combination of therapies is recommended, usually a cognitive behaviour therapy plus a modern or classic antidepressant. Two further choices of treatment should lead in the direction of a combination between medication and cognitive behaviour therapy. Thereafter, specialised treatment

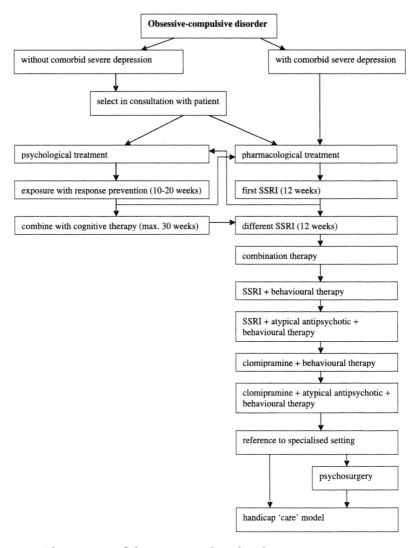

Fig. 2 The treatment of obsessive-compulsive disorder (LSR, 2003)

can be recommended or discontinuation of treatment and adoption of the handicap model.

For the psychological treatment of anxiety disorders, there is no mention whatsoever of the classic person-oriented psychotherapies. The same holds true for more contextual social interventions, non-verbal therapies, and specific nurse interventions. The arguments are clear: 'The effectiveness of these interventions has not yet been systematically studied to a sufficient extent to justify conclusions with regard to their efficacy and the durability of the effects' (LSR 2005: 82).

Mixed reactions

The guideline approach has been seriously criticised (Hutschemaekers & Smeets 2005). Here we will mention the most important criticisms of this scientific theory and its content.

1. *Unscientific* – When translating the 'evidence' into standards, the results are weighed on the basis of their 'levels of evidence' and subsequently on the basis of the size of the effects. Following this, the achieved sequence is put into the standards. The logic of this system is as follows: start with the most effective intervention, and if this does not work, choose an intervention for which the efficacy is a little smaller. Such an interpretation is not evidence-based though; there is not enough evidence to show that an intervention which has been proved to be effective can still be effective once it has been preceded by another even more effective intervention (Kampman et al. 2002).

2. *The dodo bird verdict* – Our trust in the objectivity of scientific research is too large: Research results on various therapies show that there is a high degree of covariance with the beliefs of the leading researcher (Luborsky et al. 1999). The dodo bird verdict essentially states that interventions are more effective the more the researcher expects from them. This outcome even applies to randomised double-blind studies.

3. *Effective is not the same as suitable* – Solid research according to the levels of evidence applies mostly to the effectivity of interventions and not to their suitability. Efficacy concerns the effects of the intervention under ideal circumstances, while suitability concerns the effects found in daily practice. It is mostly accepted that effective interventions are also suitable (Tanenbaum 2005). The little empirical evidence that is available clearly shows a large chasm between efficacy and suitability. For example: electroshock intervention is the most effective treatment for depression, but the majority of patients refuse this treatment option.

4. *Care means more than just reducing the symptoms* – RCT research (level 1) concentrates on the demand of reducing symptoms. However, treatments entail more than just reducing symptoms. The goals that have been set, for example, are concerned with the meaning that people attach to their symptoms, or changes in the ways they cope and manage their symptoms. Empowerment, for instance, tends to be more appreciated by patients than medications for reducing symptoms (Berg et al. 2001)

5. *Care is more than just interventions by treating disciplines* – Those disciplines not directly involved with the treatment (psychiatric nurses, social workers, vocational therapists, etc.) also have a role in mental health care, but are at a disadvantage as far as effectivity research is concerned. Aspects such as respect and dignity for clients during an

admission period or the increased value of a clinical department without a separation area are not easy to study with the RCT design. When standards are limited to the highest level of evidence, the value of these aspects will remain underexposed (Hutschemaekers & Smeets 2005).

6. *The added value of experience-based knowledge* – The last argument we will tackle here is that of the added value of experience-based knowledge (knowledge resulting from patient experiences). Experience-based knowledge is particularly valuable for questions concerning if and how an intervention should be recommended for specific client groups, or which possible relevant but not-yet charted side effects there are (Hutschemaekers 2001). This knowledge does not come to the fore as long as the focus remains on hard evidence.

Passive Roles

In light of this criticism, the results of this guideline approach of evidence-based policy are far-reaching: mental health care ends up governed by a 'positivistic' ideology that reduces care to symptom reduction. More implicit but probably even more dramatic is its vision of the roles of the professional and the client, which are reduced to an implementer of guidelines or to a receiver of care for whom certain interventions take place. Because information is available on which intervention in which setting leads to the largest reduction in symptoms, the caregiver is expected to adhere completely to the standard information. Every personal addition potentially spoils the effect. An ideal therapist therefore acts like a computer; he performs what is expected of him in an extremely competent manner. In this model, he becomes a competent implementer of procedures that have been developed by others and to which no individual clinical expertise can be added. The client is in exactly the same position because the ideal client is the one who is prepared to act according to the standard. This means no extra questions, no personal contributions, and certainly no personal opinion on what is happening. This process links up with the dominant medical perspective where clients' problems are translated into disorders that occur inside the client without him having any direct influence on the process.

Appealing Power

Despite the strong criticism on the new standard for anxiety disorders, all clients and professional organisations involved have subscribed to them. We have to ask ourselves why this is so. What has prompted professionals and patient organisations to adopt these standards? The literature suggests that normative and power elements may account for the popularity of the guideline approach (Vos et al. 2003).

First there is the clients' consent. The new standards may provide more insight into effective interventions and offer clients more opportunities to be well-prepared when entering into negotiations with their caregivers. In addition, clients may be seeing a kind of recognition in the medical approach adhered to in the standards concerning their suffering and illness. This argument has in its favour the fact that those patient organisations that are diagnosis-oriented have reacted more enthusiastically than patient organisations with a more general orientation (LSR 2005).

Equally striking is the approval by all of the professional organisations. This may have come primarily from professional societies, which are responsible for the development of these guidelines and may have strengthened their own role in the process. The position of professional societies has changed together with the new guidelines as they are now in a position to determine which interventions can be offered. In other words, part of the professional autonomy of the individual lies in their hands, and guidelines provide them with the opportunity to discipline members.

As far as the separate professional groups are concerned, there may be different arguments that play a role in each individual case. The viewpoints of psychiatrists and psychologists are the easiest to understand. Their interventions are the most prominent ones mentioned in the guidelines. Also, the dominant medical specialist perspective links up well with the dominant views within both professional groups. In this way, the guideline approach and the standards that result from this further strengthen their positions. Moreover, their professions have been now completely rehabilitated from the detrimental effects of the 1960s antipsychiatric movement. Back then, these two professional groups were by far the biggest losers in the fight for professionalisation (Hutschemaekers & Neijmeijer 1998).

The same cannot be said for psychotherapists and social workers, however. Their interventions have not been included in the standards, meaning that they are now the biggest losers and their position is being crushed ever further (Hutschemaekers & Van den Staak, in press). It is not purely by chance that both these professional groups, as proponents of the process approach in mental health care rather than adherents of the medical model, were previously (at the time of the antipsychiatric movement) the bigger winners in the fight between these professions (Blok 2004). Why, then, did they approve the new standards? Was this due to a lack of knowledge on their part, or to an extreme state of demoralisation that resulted in an insufficient restoration of critical abilities? Apparently, the new standards include a number of positive incentives for these professionals. The introduction of the standards allows for the development of different relationships between professionals, the political world, and the general public (Timmerans & Kolker 2004). According to Freidson, it could be argued that the standards are a weapon used in the fight for professional autonomy and against the first (market) and second (bureaucratic) logic (Freidson 2001). In that case, the guideline approach of evidence-based policy could also help in the fight for the power of professionals.

The question remains whether the price paid for the guideline approach is not excessively high. Our viewpoint is that this is indeed the case. This is even more true when considering that evidence-based policy used in a heuristic way could offer professionals many opportunities for taking their own professional responsibility.

The Heuristic Approach

The meaning of the term 'evidence-based' described above is completely contrary to the roots of the concept. The term originally comes from the field of education. In the mid-1980s, evidence-based medicine (EBM) was introduced at the McMaster Medical School (Canada) as the name for a new educational method (EBM working group 1992). According to its developers, EBM is a learning method that enables doctors-in-training to work according to the latest scientific insights without having to delve into scientific journals for hours every day. Reading article after article too easily leads to the idea that science only deals with large groups of patients and does not include specific information for the one patient they are treating at present. EBM was developed in order to encourage caregivers to take a more active approach towards attaining knowledge (Sackett et al. 2000).

This didactic or heuristic evidence-based approach is an elaboration of the principles that have been described in the authoritative standard work 'Clinical Epidemiology' (Fletcher et al. 1991). The most accepted definition of evidence-based medicine stems from this work and dates from 2000: 'EBM is the integration of [the] best research evidence with clinical expertise and patient values' (Sackett et al. 2000: 1). Above all, EBM is a practice whereby professionals search and consider various sorts of knowledge, subsequently applying what they have learned in specific situations and finally evaluating the results. EBM is thus merely a heuristic tool that can help combine different sources of knowledge.

The EBM heuristic is divided into five steps. In the first step, the problem that has been found in daily practice is formulated into an answerable question according to a fixed system. The second step consists of searching out and selecting the relevant knowledge. The results of this search operation are then considered for their scientific value, impact and applicability in daily practice. In step four, the decision is taken of whether or not to apply the measures in light of the clinical expertise and the applicability for this particular patient, taking into account his personal wishes. In step five, the results of the treatment steps taken are evaluated. We will now explain these steps in more detail:

1. EBM starts with a problem that occurs in daily practice, mostly in the diagnosis or treatment of a specific patient. EBM provides a sort of helping hand to translate the problem at stake into an answerable question. In other words, a general problem is turned into a case study. This appears to be simple in theory, but it is not. Inexperienced caregivers turn out to mostly formulate general questions. Sackett refers to these as background questions (Sackett et al. 2000). These concern, for example, general symptoms of a disease or therapy, e.g., how often does depression go hand in hand with diabetes. While it is true that these questions are important, they are not specific to the patient for whom the question was formulated. The more the caregiver gains clinical experience, the more he is able to formulate 'foreground questions' (Sackett et al. 2000). These questions are quite focused on the treatment details of the particular patient. For example: is cognitive behavioural therapy more effective than medication in reducing symptoms in the long term in a diabetic patient with depression? A well-formulated foreground question will lead to an answer that has direct consequences on the treatment.

    Foreground questions are arranged according to the PICO system (which stands for patient population, intervention, comparison, and outcome). Adhering to a PICO system enables professionals to clearly define what they want to know: formulation of relevant patient characteristics, the intervention, any possible alternative treatment methods and desired outcomes. These outcomes may be a reduction in the number and seriousness of the symptoms, or they may relate to such concepts as empowerment or a person's ability to cope with daily activities, etc. The PICO system enables a unique problem to be described in such a way that it is possible to subsequently search the literature.

2. Searching and selecting existing knowledge. The starting point of EBM is that the (mostly published) knowledge of others can contribute to the solution of the formulated problem. Within the EBM tradition, the answer is usually first searched for in the jungle of the literature, and mostly in large databases such as Medline, Psychlite, or the Cochrane library. The question does not usually concern whether or not there is information on the problem concerned but how this can be retrieved. The PICO system described above can offer a helping hand in this process. The four elements included in the question of patient population, intervention, alternative intervention, and outcomes are all items that can be used as search terms in an existing database. The four components can be looked for separately by doing a broad search and the results subsequently linked up. The PICO system, as it were, is a cross-section of four collections.

    In theory, it is possible that the literature does not provide the answers to the questions that have been posed. This is more often the case when the 'body of evidence' within a specific area is more limited. In this case, other resources will have to be consulted, such as a colleague with more experience on the matter. However, the developers of EBM argue that the main reason for not being able to find answers in the literature is that a question has been either too broadly or too narrowly formulated.

3. Evaluating the information and checking for applicability. The EBM method requires a lot of time to evaluate the information found. This reminds us of the old adage: just because something has been written down and published does not mean it is true. The found evidence is analysed and evaluated according to very precise criteria. Finally, the level of evidence is determined. Attention is paid to dates and the prioritising of the latest information. Manuals and guidelines are by definition out of date. Sackett et al. (2000) provide the following important advice: 'burn your textbooks'.

    During the process of analysis and evaluation, the results that have been found are translated so that they can be used for the original problem. A number of statistical techniques are used in order to determine the chances for effective intervention that has been examined and chosen for this specific client.

4. Deciding on the application by integrating the newly acquired knowledge with the professional's own clinical expertise (experience in daily practice) and the values and/or experiences of the client (patient's experience). The caregiver makes an estimate of the applicability of the intervention for a particular patient on the basis of his own clinical expertise. He does this by explicitly stating his expertise and opinions. Sackett then proposes that individual clinical expertise and patient values and experiences be translated in terms of chances. These chances should be brought together and reported in one coefficient (Sackett et al. 2000: 123-129). There are still a few snags as far as the actual implementation is concerned, but the underlying principle is clear: scientific evidence, experience-based knowledge and clinical expertise should be joined to support the decision that always falls under the responsibility of the professional caregiver.

5. Evaluation of the results. PICO helps to explain the aim of the intervention, and explicit treatment goals are essential in order to determine the result. Ideally, on the basis of the collected evidence, it should become clear which results can be expected within which period of time, as well as the measuring instruments used. These are the most important parameters for measuring the results. One characteristic for a good EBM approach is that the caregiver ensures this result is achieved. In turn, this provides leads that can be used in evaluating the intervention, and if necessary show the way to adaptations in the treatment.

In sum, EBM is a heuristic that professionals can use in order to tackle clinical problems via the systematic integration of scientific evidence, individual clinical expertise, and patients' values and experiences. Although it is true that EBM does make a statement on the scientific merits of interventions based on the criteria for the level of evidence, the scientific evidence is only one of the aspects involved in the decision that ultimately lies with the individual professional.

Learning Professionals

The EBM heuristic is widely applicable for various questions and problems that occur in the day-to-day treatment and care of patients. While searching for and using scientific evidence is, at first glance, more suitable for use with professions holding a sizeable 'body of evidence', it is clear from daily practice that other professional groups such as social workers and nurses also benefit from this concept (Geddes & Harrison 1997; Scholte & Hutschemaekers 2004; Cox et al. 2004). This is in fact logical, because EBM is primarily a practice of the systematic analysis of problems that occur in daily clinical practice.

The evidence-based heuristic and guideline approaches do agree on several points. They are congruent on the point of creating a distance from a care practice that is dominated by an attitude of 'just carrying on', intuition, power by force of habit, or hierarchy. In both approaches, the intention is to improve care by using scientific evidence. Their analysis of scientific evidence is also identical in terms of levels of evidence. In both approaches, the main concern is with care that is evidence-based as much as possible.

However, in a number of aspects, the heuristic approach is directly opposite to the evidence-based guideline approach. The departure point of the heuristic approach lies in a problem occurring in daily practice (bottom-up), whereas the guideline approach begins with the evidence itself and moves from that point towards practice (top-down). The value of the 'evidence' is more absolute in the guideline approach than in the heuristic approach. In the latter, research evidence is integrated into the individual expertise of the professional involved and the personal experience of the client. In the heuristic approach the professional is primarily seeking a solution to a problem, in the guideline approach he is just the implementer.

This difference is fundamental when looked at from the perspective of professionalisation (Hutschemaekers 2001). The quality of professional performance is not only better when new skills are learned and adopted, but also and perhaps even more so, by reflection and awareness of one's own performance. According to Schön (1983: 49-69), the simple question 'Why am I doing this?' encourages explanation and a systematic approach to existing practices. The following question would be, 'Am I doing what is best?' This process is characterised by the fact that the caregiver formulates both the questions and answers himself. This individual activity is typical for each experience relating to 'sense of mastery'.

This vision of the individual activity links up directly with a report made by the Dutch Health Council (Gezondheidsraad 2000) on the implementation of standards. At the request of the Minister of Health, the council concentrated on the question of how the implementation of standards could be improved. The answer was: 'Minister, you are really asking the wrong question'. The implementation of standards suggests that professionals should change their behaviour through specific top-down activities. This will not work. Instead, the following question should be asked: 'How do professionals learn?' As soon as professionals learn, they search out available knowledge and consequently arrive at the existing evidence.

From Answer to Question

Evidence-based policy often takes the form of a set of rules, giving the primacy of the science. Care improves as professionals adhere more strictly to the guidelines of the science. The result is that professionals change into honest implementers of evidence-based interventions. Everything that the professional does on his own initiative should be seen as a disturbance. In an ideal future, the computer and the robot will have taken over all of the tasks from the professional.

The heuristic perspective on evidence-based policy is very different from the above. Here too, much value is attached to scientific evidence, although the relationship between professional and science is defined differently. Care improves as soon as professionals ask questions more often on the 'why' of their interventions. The more they ask why, the more often they find possible alternatives. The evidence-based approach offers a helping hand so that the questions can be asked in such a way that three sources of knowledge can be consulted: scientific knowledge, clinical experience of the professional and personal experience of the client. Ultimately, it is again the professional who has to decide what happens. The choice belongs to his core competences, for which he carries responsibility and which he must account for.

Evidence-based heuristics link up well with modern learning theories and opinions on the subject of professionalisation. However, this does not distract from the fact that the heuristic approach too has limitations. The approach is stronger as goals and intervention are explained better. It is also true that the heuristic approach works best for those interventions that are not very strongly connected to their socio-cultural context, i.e., those interventions that can been studied under experimental conditions (according to the RCT design). The more the effectiveness of an intervention is restricted to a specific context, the less that intervention can help to solve problems in other contexts. The EBM heuristic also has limitations for the assessment of practice knowledge and experience-based knowledge. These sources of knowledge are explicitly conceptualised by Sackett et al. (2000), but the way in which this knowledge should be evaluated and used within the EBM heuristic is too vague and so complicated that it is hard to perform in daily practice. We therefore believe that the EBM heuristic should further elaborate on this point.

In our opinion, the warnings the literature has given on the possible harmful effects of this ideology for professionals and clients are right. Whether the consequences will be as far-reaching as has been suggested is questionable. Criticism on the guideline approach is widespread (Hutschemaekers & Smeets 2005). Some even talk of a new value-based approach emerging (Fulford 2003). Evidence on its own cannot possibly steer the care practice; first and foremost, the values of different treatment goals have to be made more explicit. This point concerns such questions as: do we want to achieve a minimum chance of failure or a maximum chance of success? (Berg et al. 2001)

Does the same judgement apply to the products of the evidence-based guideline approach, and will the guidelines always be at odds with the evidence-based method? Strictly and theoretically speaking, this will be the case, according to Sackett et al. (2000). This is due to the fact that guidelines are already out of date as soon they appear, and could give the impression that the professional is merely an implementer. In reality, a guideline can be used reliably. As soon as a caregiver and a client come to the conclusion that the solution to a specific problem should be translated into a reduction of symptoms, the guideline can be a valuable instrument in determining which interventions should be applied and in which order. In this case, the guideline is used heuristically. The developers of the multidisciplinary standard for anxiety disorders discussed in this chapter argue explicitly for such a well-reasoned use (Hutschemaekers & Smeets 2005).

Our conclusion is that, in the end, the evidence-based guideline ideology is perhaps the biggest danger when placed in the hands of those professionals who are the least prepared to discuss their performance. The professional who is unable to question his clinical practice cannot benefit from knowledge and experience that has been derived and collected from others. From this perspective, we may be able to redefine the main problem with the professionals of Chestnut Lodge in the Osheroff case. Their real problem was not that they did not treat their patient with medication, but that they did not raise any questions about the efficacy of their own psychotherapeutic treatment.

Note

1. Chestnut Lodge was the home of the antipsychiatric movement in the US in the 1960s. On the basis of his experiences there, Foudraine wrote the bestseller Not Made of Wood (1971).

Societal Neurosis in Health Care

Margo Trappenburg

In 1994, Michael Power, a chartered accountant and lecturer in accounting and finance at the London School of Economics, published an intriguing essay, entitled The Audit Explosion. Power argued that the growing multitude of audit procedures had changed the nature of service delivery. People and organisations that were consistently being audited – such as hospitals, schools, water companies, laboratories, and various industries – start thinking differently about their own activities; they start looking at their work from an auditor's point of view. They focus on the measurable and quantifiable aspects of their work. Auditors generally do not see what is going on in daily practice, they do not sit in the class room, do not visit hospital wards, and do not read master theses written by students. Instead they evaluate the organisation's plans, programs, and evaluations; they tend to monitor systems of control, they look at the paper world created by the organisation for auditing purposes.

Auditing, according to Power, has developed into 'policing of policing'. An organisation that wants to survive an audit has to invest in reporting, monitoring, and policing, rather than in improving performance. Unfortunately, the audit explosion has not led to more trust in service delivery. Instead, there seems to be a 'regress of mistrust'. If those engaged in service delivery cannot be trusted, why should one trust the experts, managers, and accountants involved in policing them? Ultimately "the performances of auditors and inspectors will themselves be subjected to audit" (Power 1994: 13). This regress of mistrust may have something to do with the fact that the audit explosion has brought about "a shift from professions the public trusts more – such as doctors, police and teachers, to a profession the public trusts less (the accountants) at the instigation of a profession the public trusts least (the politicians)". (Power 1994: 35).

Onora O'Neill has made similar observations and complaints in her BBC lectures on trust (O'Neill 2002). Similar observations were also made by the British political philosopher Grahame Lock in an essay about the demise of the Netherlands. In Locke's phraseology the quest for ever more audits, control, and accountability has turned into some sort of disease, that can be called societal neurosis or hyper-rationality. Lock describes the phenomenon as follows:

> Just like the neurotic who washes his hands a thousand times a day, our hyperrational society, under the political disguise of so-called responsibility,

cannot stop producing ever more refined instruments to measure and control itself a thousand times a day. (Lock 2005: 207)

Power, O'Neill, and Lock seem to have discovered an important insight. However, they tend to focus on general trends in society. In this chapter I would like to investigate this phenomenon close up by focusing on one particular policy sector, i.e., health care in one specific country, i.e., the Netherlands. By doing so, I hope to achieve a better understanding of the underlying logic that leads to societal neurosis or the audit explosion. I also hope that an in-depth analysis may give us some clues to how to put a stop to this audit explosion, or – put more appropriately in this chapter on health care – whether and how societal neurosis can ever be cured. Building on the work by Tonkens (Tonkens 1999 and 2003), I will describe the developments in Dutch health care, starting with the democratisation movement in the 1970s and concluding in the full-blown societal neurosis of the 21st century. In the last section of this chapter, I will reflect on a possible cure for this (hopefully not lethal) disease.

The First Stage of Societal Neurosis: A Call for Patient Rights and Institutional Democracy

The seeds of societal neurosis can probably be traced back to the 1960s and 1970s, an era in which a large part of the population turned against authority figures representing "the establishment" including teachers, mayors, policemen, politicians, and doctors. It remains an open question whether the seeds of democratisation could have evolved into something other than an audit explosion, hyper-rationality, or societal neurosis. I would like to think that they could have, but social scientists cannot turn back the clock and start their social experiments afresh.

In health care, the revolution of the 1960s started in psychiatric wards. You may remember the movie ONE FLEW OVER THE CUCKOO'S NEST (1975), based on the 1962 novel by Ken Kesey. Former prison inmate, Randle P. McMurphy, as played by Jack Nicholson enters a psychiatric ward and challenges the authority of Nurse Ratched. Health care social movements have questioned medical authority, either because they did not respect authority in general or because they had witnessed various forms of abuse of that authority, such as corporate doctors who hide information regarding conditions in the asbestos industry, or medical researchers who conduct dangerous medical experiments involving unsuspecting patients (Brown & Zavestoski 2005). Despite this origin of resistance against medical authority there has also always been a close, almost natural alliance between patients and doctors. Patients who want to be cured need doctors, doctors have been trained to take their patients' interests seriously and generally earn an income by doing so. Governments who establish a goal of reducing medical resources usually meet with fierce resistance from both patients and doctors (Blank & Burau 2004; cf. also Freeman 2000).

Oudenampsen (1999), Rijkschroeff (1989), Stüssgen (1997) and Verkaar (1991) have analysed the origins of the patient movement in the Netherlands. According to Verkaar, patient organisations in those days employed four strategies:

1. the substitute care strategy, directed at the replacement of regular care by other forms of treatment offered by the patient organisation (think of Alcoholics Anonymous which organises group sessions and group support as an alternative to the regular counselling agencies for substance abuse, or of patient groups that favour alternative treatment);
2. the protest strategy, aimed at the abolition of certain parts of the health care system (e.g., the Dutch organisation for psychiatric patients, the Cliëntenbond, was opposed to psychiatric care in general and electroshock therapy in particular; following the ideology of the anti-psychiatry movement they argued that many mental patients should not be viewed as patients in the first place because their conditions could be viewed as an appropriate response to a sick society);
3. the improvement strategy, aimed at transforming the regular health care system; and
4. the additional care strategy, which – as the word suggests – was meant to supplement the regular care offered by the medical system.

The government, almost from the very beginning, looked upon the patient movement favourably (Nederland and Duyvendak 2004; Nederland, Duyvendak and Brugman 2003). Of course, this warm welcome may have been due to a true commitment to the goals and interests of the patient movement. However, it may also have had something to do with the fact that the government had been engaged in a frustrating battle with medical specialists over their incomes (Trappenburg & De Groot 2001). Politicians may have seen the patient movement as a possible ally against the medical elite. The first two strategies employed by the patient movement seemed truly promising in this respect.

The first strategy (opting out of the health care system and turning to self-help instead) seemed to concur with money-saving government concepts such as 'family care' and 'neighbourhood care' instead of more expensive professional help. This may have been one of the reasons why patient organisations were readily included in the policy-making process. Patient organisations were granted representation in the sickness fund council and the National Council for Public Health. They were asked to regroup in regional platforms, which were to be paid by the provinces. These regional platforms could delegate patient representatives to meetings with the local governments in which matters such as provisions for the handicapped and community care were being discussed (Oudenampsen 1999). Rijkschroeff describes how representatives of the patient movement were overwhelmed by government requests to participate in all sorts of advisory bodies, councils, committees, and advisory meetings with the government. 'Once you get in, it seems that one participation activity leads to another'. (Rijkschroeff 1989: 13).

The second strategy employed by patient organisations (which aims to redefine the status of patients and the abolition of certain kinds of treatments) may have contributed to the introduction of legislation about patient rights, such as the Law on the Medical Treatment Contract (the WGBO, which codified principles such as the right to be informed about one's medical treatment, the principle of consent and the right to refuse consent) and the Law on Forced Admittance to Pyschiatric Hospitals, the BOPZ. The BOPZ replaced the former law on the mentally insane, which had stated that psychiatric patients could be put away against their wishes if this was for their own good. Under the BOPZ regime, patients could not be locked up in a psychiatric ward unless they were a danger to themselves or others.

Those patients who were still committed to a psychiatric hospital (against their wishes or voluntarily, because their conditions were too serious to live outside the confines of a hospital ward) strove for institutional democracy. Client and patient councils were installed, at first in mental health care, but later also in homes for the elderly and homes for the mentally disabled (usually the mentally retarded inmates of these homes were represented by their parents).

In 1996, a law that forced health care institutions to establish a client council strengthened the position of these client councils. Institutions that had never had a client council before (hospitals and organisations for short-term out-patient psychiatric care) were required to establish one as well. The client councils were given a voice in important issues concerning care. They went beyond merely dealing with the daily lives of patients within the facility (food, atmosphere, outings, parties and so on), they also became involved in discussions concerning such complicated issues as mergers with other institutions, management's vision on the future, new building projects, complicated financial reports, and so on.

In addition to the law on institutional democracy in health care (the WMCZ), patients were given the legal right to complain about their health care professionals to a complaints committee.

All these laws emphasise that patients have rights and claims against their doctors, nurses, care institutions, and hospitals, thus picturing professionals and professional institutions not as allies in a common fight against disease, but as actors who have their own interests and their own agendas, who must be compelled to listen to their patients and clients. All these measures (the codification of patient rights, the representation of patients in advisory councils and institutional councils and the right to complain) seemed to turn patients against health care professionals.

Many political scientists have described the phenomenon of 'iron triangles' or 'policy networks'. Decisions with regard to certain policy areas are often taken in 'policy communities' consisting of powerful pressure groups, advisory councils, civil servants and politicians who feel close to the involved pressure groups. Thus, in many countries, agricultural policy used to be made in a policy community dominated by farmer pressure groups, and civil servants and politicians with agricultural backgrounds. Social security policy was made in policy communities dominated by unions, employers associations and civil servants and politicians with a background in either one of these two groups. Likewise, health policy used to be made in a policy community dominated by health professionals' interest groups (cf. Van den Berg & Molleman 1977, Smith 1993, Rhodes 1997, Marsh 1998). Politicians have not limited themselves to reserved participation in these policy communities. They have time and again also tried to undermine these communities by employing other types of civil servants (cf. De Haan & Duyvendak 2002) or by recruiting and appointing other politicians (who would not feel any connection to the department they were chairing, because they did not have a background in farming, the workers' movement or the health sector), for instance. Politicians have also managed to undermine policy communities by opening them up for other interest groups by, for example, inviting consumer interest groups in the agricultural community. Thus patient-consumer groups were invited into the health policy community, on the implicit condition that they would not serve as allies to the medical profession (Kjaer 2004). This seems to have been the case in the Dutch health care sector.

As noted above, the Dutch patient movement (or rather: the patient organisations) did not just employ negative strategies against the medical profession, but they also sought to improve, supplement, and support current health care, and these strategies (in terms of the aforementioned analysis by Verkaar involving the improvement and additional care strategies) seemed to warrant much more co-operation with health care professionals. However, during the 1990s, these strategies would gradually be curbed and forced to go in another direction. Instead of fostering the natural coalition between patients and professionals, these two strategies (like the oppositional strategies discussed before) would be turned into weapons against professionals as well. An early sign of this phenomenon was the so-called Quality Law, introduced in 1996. This law required that care providers develop a quality system and produce annual quality reports, which were to be submitted to patient organisations and health insurers, who would then have to judge the care providers' attempts to improve the quality of care (cf. Casparie et al. 2001).

The alleged conflict of interests between professionals on the one hand, and patients and their organisations on the other, was only exacerbated with the new plans for the marketisation of health care, which will be discussed in the next section.

The Second Stage of Societal Neurosis: The Quest for High-Quality Care on the Cheap

During the 1980s and early 1990s, politicians in European countries interested in health care were mostly busy finding ways to contain costs. In the words of health care policy expert Richard Freeman: 'Beginning at the end of the 1970s, an epidemic of reform swept the health systems of Western Europe'. (Freeman 2000: 66). In the past, health care policy had been very consensual. Equal and universal access suited both doctors, patients, employers and taxpayers, that is "both users and providers and those who ultimately paid for it." (Freeman 2000: 77). Since the 1980s, however, all this has changed. The downward pressure on fees and other health expenses led to the introduction of managers in hospitals, who would try to meet targets, cut back on resources, and interfere with clinical autonomy. Of course, there had been health care managers in the past, but their powers were always limited. Traditional health care managers were inclined to solve problems and maintain their organisations, rather than institute major changes (Harrison 1999). But with the introduction of 'the cost containment imperative', managers were given much more influence in the goings on of health care organisations.

Similarly, the impact of politics in the health care systems grew substantially. Politicians consciously aimed to reform their health care systems. Since it did not seem politically viable to boldly announce that health care was just going to get for the worse, for both doctors and patients alike, governments in many countries tried to depict their reform policy as essentially motivated by the patient interests (Freeman 2000). Hence, the cutbacks in health care were accompanied by the introduction of patient councils, patient charters, and endless procedures for quality control and cost containment under the heading of New Public Management. Patient advocacy groups seem to have been manipulated to foist health care reforms on an unwilling public (Dibben & Higgins 2004, also Freeman 2000).

Let us take a closer look at what happened in the Netherlands.

The health care system in the Netherlands was neither a tax-financed national health service (as in the UK or Scandinavian countries) nor an outright, premium-based social insurance system (as the Belgian or German systems). Until 2006 the Dutch health care system consisted of three layers. Long-term institutional care (in a psychiatric hospital, a geriatric ward, or an institute for the mentally disabled) was financed by means of a social insurance system, which covered the entire population. Less-expensive care for chronically ill, elderly, or handicapped patients was also included here. 'Ordinary' hospital care, visits to general practitioners, midwives, and various other provisions broadly classified as 'cures', were financed differently for different segments of the population. This second layer of the Dutch health care system consisted of two parts. Roughly two-thirds of the population was legally obliged to pay income-based health care premiums. Health care funds provided cures or care in kind for these citizens. The remaining one-third of the population (mostly those with higher incomes) could choose a private health insurer. There were some elements of solidarity built into the private insurance section of the second layer. Private insurers had to offer less-healthy clients whom they might otherwise refuse a so-called standard package. These high-risk clients were required to pay high premiums for this standard package, but these premiums in no way fully covered their health care costs. The healthier privately insured clients had to pay a solidarity bonus on top of their premiums to make up for the losses incurred by private insurers as a result of their chronically ill or otherwise extremely expensive clients. The third layer in the Dutch health care system was very small and consisted mostly of non-essential medical provisions, which people could do without or might choose to pay out of pocket, should they desire to.

How could one reduce expenses in this kind of a system?

In actual political practice, three different policy instruments were employed to reduce health care costs, all of which could be classified as supply-side instruments.

1. Everything that could be budgeted was budgeted (hospital budgets, budgets for certain operations, macro health care budgets).
2. Medical doctors were strongly encouraged to make and follow professional guidelines. Following a 1991 report by the Health Care Council, in which the council argued that there were far too many differences between doctors about what kind of treatment or medicine should be prescribed under what conditions, the profession was asked to make medical practice more 'evidence-based'.
3. Certain provisions were taken from the collective insurance health care packages because they were not considered to be evidence-based, or because they were not meant to remedy a truly pathological condition (e.g., physiotherapy was deemed to be not evidence-based and involuntary infertility, albeit it very tragic, was not considered a handicap or a disease, hence fertility treatments were largely thrown out of the collective insurance packages).

These three policy instruments were very effective; the percentage of the gross national product spent on health care rose from 7.0% in 1975 to 8.7% in 1998 (Blank & Burau 2004), which was a very moderate increase, for example, compared to the US (from 7.2% to 12.9% in the same period).

However, despite this apparent success in actual policy, and despite the fact that the OECD considers supply-side measures a much more effective way of cost containment than demand-side measures (Blank & Burau 2004), the political rhetoric tended to move in another direction. In 1986, the Dutch government had installed an ad hoc committee chaired by Philips business tycoon Wisse Dekker to consider the future of the health care system. The Dekker Committee in its 1987 report argued that Dutch health care could benefit from a system of managed competition, in which health care insurers would have to play an important role in guarding the quality of care by deciding whether or not to include one or another health care provider in the insurance packages they offered. Thus, health care providers who did not meet professional standards or who charged too much for their services, would be disqualified by the insurers and lose their clientele. The idea of making (mildly) profit-oriented insurers assume the health care costs has never really left the political agenda since the Dekker Committee's reports, although their plans were not implemented as such.

In addition to the Dekker proposals, government ministers felt that, if a system of managed competition were adopted, there had to be a larger role not just for the insurers but also for the various patient organisations. They should be allowed to evaluate medical performance and advise insurers about whom to contract under what conditions. However, in order to be up to this particular task, patient organisations first had to be strengthened and professionalised. Patient advocacy groups have been explicitly encouraged to merge with consumer groups and to behave as consumers, in order to perform the role they should play under a new public management regime. Patient organisations were invited to participate in top conferences on the quality of medical care, they were asked to reflect about and discuss reform plans with the government. In order to be able to fulfil this task patient organisations were heavily subsidised by the so-called Patient Fund (introduced in 1996). Many organisations were newly created, while many other organisations could afford to hire professional staff. At the national level, the NPCF (the National Platform for Patient and Consumer Organisations) developed into a large organisation, staffed by a number of employees.

Patient organisations were strongly encouraged to fall back on two strategies that they were familiar with: Focus on the improvement and possible expansion of regular medical care. However, they were no longer allowed to use these strategies in close collaboration with medical professionals. It was somehow taken for granted that medical professionals would not be willing to think about alternative treatments or improved care on their own. It was accepted that they very much needed material incentives and external controls. Patient organisations and insurers were the ones who could provide this, according to the government. The ongoing development towards evidence-based medicine and the traditional forms of disciplinary control within the medical profession (disciplinary law and the health care inspection) were deemed to be not enough to guarantee quality care.

Henceforth, professionals would have to become more open and transparent regarding their actions, they would have to admit mistakes, register their every move, and cluster their movements into a multitude of indicators involving, for instance, the number of patients suffering from decubitus in their hospital, the number of operations which went slightly wrong, the amount of pain suffered by patients after their operations, the number of high-tech medical instruments in their hospitals and so on and so forth. Representatives of patient organisations and health insurers would then compare the scores of hospitals, hospital departments or even individual doctors and judge performance based on these comparisons.

The almost infinite amount of storage space on the Internet has made it possible to save a multitude of lists of performance indicators and the professional scores given these indicators. Not only patient organisations and health insurers can use this information; individual patients can also access it as well.

Many professionals obviously end up complaining about the administrative and bureaucratic overloads thrust upon them, but these complaints always sound slightly suspicious because a professional who does not want transparency obviously has something hide.

Recent (2004-2005) reform plans, launched by Health Minister Hoogervorst, but still very much inspired by the Dekker report, expected a scenario of health care providers continuously busy delivering data on the quality of care they provide, and a coalition of eager insurers and well-informed patient organisations who decide whom to contract at what price for what kind of services (cf. TK 27807, no. 22 and TK 28439, no. 7). Moreover, Hoogervorst emphasised that the Quality Law will be further amended in the future, to make it even stricter on care providers (EK 29 763, no. 22).

Societal neurosis thus starts with democratisation and then takes a turn for the worse via new public management reforms that involve bureaucratic marketisation.

The Third Stage of Societal Neurosis: Hyper-Control

Under the new health care system, health insurers and patient organisations will have to monitor and control the performance of doctors and other medical professionals. However, individual patients (or, as the market rhetoric would prefer: individual consumers or clients) will basically not choose doctors or hospitals. They will instead have to first choose a health insurer. This means that they will have to be able to compare the insurance packages offered by the various health insurers. Ideally they should be able to compare the prices, the quality of the total package, and the insurance conditions of different insurers such as the percentage of co-payments. Hence, it is paramount that the insurers provide information about their performance histories and their future policies, like medical professionals had to do before. These data will have to be evaluated – like the medical performance data – by patient organisations, but they are certainly not the only ones who will be called upon to monitor the insurers. The Dutch Senate recently organised a meeting with relevant actors involved in the implementation of the new health insurance system. During this meeting Rogier van Boxtel, chairman of the board of directors of a large health insurance company, neatly summed up the institutions that will monitor his organisation in the future: monitoring by patient organisations, but also supervision by the Financial Market's Authority (AFM), the Dutch central bank (DNB), the Dutch Authority on Competition (NMA), and the future Health Care Authority (Zorgautoriteit, the present CTG).

Eric Fischer, of the Insurers Federation, expressed his concern about all these monitoring and control authorities. In his opinion, these organisations were staffed by policymakers, that is by creative people who continuously need to demonstrate their worth and thus continue to invent ever better, more advanced, and more refined monitoring methods. Fischer believes that there should at least be some time left to actually do one's work (EK 29762/29763, proceedings of a hearing, 29 April 2005, 12).

There does not seem to be much chance that these complaints will be resolved, however. Hoogervorst has emphasised that the health insurers definitely have to be controlled and monitored by these various authorities (EK 29763, 90). Moreover, they will have to provide data to the Institute for Public Health and Environment (the RIVM), which will organise surveys in order to acquire data on patient satisfaction, that can subsequently be published on the internet so that it can be used by (potential) clients (EK 29763, 95).

Given the fact that they were the ones who advocated transparency and comparable data with regard to medical practices, it would be inconsistent for insurers to argue that insurers themselves should not have to conform to the same types of rules and regulations.

Meanwhile, we can sum up an impressive list of tasks for the patient organisations:
- they must staff client councils if the patients of homes and hospitals do not volunteer for these councils (staffing these councils has been a problem almost from the beginning and still is, cf. Rijkschroeff 1989; Casparie et al. 2001);
- they must monitor the quality reports of the health care organisations and must continue to do so in the future when the law will become even more exacting;

- they must participate in all sorts of meetings with policy makers on the local, regional and national level;
- they must monitor the performance of care providers (nursing homes, hospitals, homes for the mentally retarded, general practitioners), and discuss what to do with this information with health insurers;
- they must monitor the performance of health insurers, in order to be able to advise their members and other patients on insurance packages and optimum treatments.

It is not surprising that the representatives of patient organisations invariably react to new proposals by demanding extra money from the government. They cannot perform all these tasks with a bunch of volunteers, they need a highly educated, trained and paid staff to meet all these demands. Hence, an important element in the Minister of Health's new plans is the empowerment of patient organisations in order to enable them to perform their ever-expanding roles (EK 29 763, 13; TK 27 807 no. 22). The special fund which distributes subsidy money to patient organisations (the former Patient fund) will receive a large budget. However, this money does not come cost-free – there are strings attached to this subsidy package. Patient organisations will have to show how they intend to perform their new tasks and will have to prove that they actually did so afterwards. The minister intends to produce "as much results as possible for care users". And here we definitely enter the phase of hyper-control. The patient organisations will not only have to spend a huge amount of time, money and effort monitoring the quality of care, and evaluating professionals' and insurers' performances, they will have to become equally transparent themselves about their own plans and performances. The special fund that distributes the government's money to patient advocacy groups has drawn up a complicated set of rules and guidelines involving performance areas and indicators for patient organisations (cf. for the new rules and regulations).

And there is no escaping it. If a patient organisation decides to disregard the special fund and the government's stipulations and look for money elsewhere, for example, in the pharmaceutical industry, it would be suspected of having compromised its objectivity and of being 'unduly influenced' by the industry. Recently, the special patient organisation subsidy fund organised research concerning money flows between the pharmaceutical industry and patient organisations (DGV 2005). The researchers found that a lot of patient organisations had indeed received money from the pharmaceutical industry in one form or another, and they were appalled by the absence of policies in many patient organisations that dealt with this subject. Some patient organisations were totally opposed to pharmaceutical industry sponsorship. Others saw no problem whatsoever with any form of sponsorship. The vast majority thought sponsorship was potentially warranted under certain conditions, which many of them apparently tried to formulate on a case by case basis (Shall we ask pharmaceutical company X to donate money for our conference? What if they want to be present then and distribute leaflets or gadgets? Do you think it would be all right to have an article written by a researcher connected to the pharmaceutical industry in our journal? Do you think we should charge them for that? Or shall we send the article to our advisory board and let a doctor referee it? And so on.) Most patient organisations prefer this modus operandi. They want to remain autonomous and make their own policies in this area, as in many others as well. The researchers are highly suspicious of this approach, however. They argue that patient organisations should come together and work out one code of conduct concerning sponsorship. This ought to be a code with strict conditions, in order to minimise the chances that individual organisations interpret the code as they see fit. This code should at the very least apply to all organisations receiving public money from the special fund. The researchers add ominously: "A code of behaviour without active supervision on compliance is mere window dressing. Therefore, conditions should be created and a means should be developed to monitor pharmaceutical companies and patient organisations to ensure they abide by their code of conduct. It must also be possible to impose sanctions, preferably performed by an existing organisation" (DGV 2005, 37).

The director of the special fund thought it might be a good idea if the pharmaceutical industry simply donated a lump sum of money, which could then be redistributed to the patient organisations by an independent organisation (Bouma & Brandt 2005).

No doubt the day will come when someone will suggest that we monitor the performance of the special fund that distributes the money to patient organisations, and then yet another organisation that evaluates the way the special fund is being monitored by its supervising agency and at some point or other, as Grahame Lock writes, we will realise that we are like the neurotic, checking and monitoring, washing our hands a thousand times a day (cf. also Engelen 2005).

Societal Neurosis: Can It Be Cured?

It is not easy to develop a cure for societal neurosis. Every individual actor who protests against transparency, performance indicators and close supervision is thus immediately under suspicion. Probably he or she has something to hide, he or she cannot live up to the performance criteria, is ashamed, and therefore does not want to confront a supervising authority.

An organisation that protests against supervision and transparency will not only have to face potentially angry policy makers and controllers, it will also risk a lot of negative publicity, because many journalists will sense a cover up and will do an investigation to unearth the organisation's secrets. Such journalistic scrutiny might even be worse than the controlling procedure by a regular supervising agency. Hence, an organisation that wants to address the ongoing societal neurosis would have to orchestrate its own publicity, it would have to invest a lot of time in talking to journalists, explaining how the administrative burdens are piling up and then hoping that journalists understand and sympathise with their stories. This is a risky strategy indeed because inevitably things do go wrong in every organisation. People are fallible, mistakes and accidents happen and the seemingly sympathetic journalist might decide to change his story and investigate further. It is not surprising that many organisations simply go along with the demands of modern times. Imagine a modern hospital or health insurance director confronting his staff: 'We have to be open, transparent, and accountable, folks, and we are going to employ two new administrative policymakers who will see to it that we are; but they cannot do it alone! They will need your help. Please register and monitor your every move; make a daily routine of it. Fill in your blue forms, and don't ever forget to submit the pink forms on time. It is paramount that we survive the upcoming supervision and quality control procedures'.

In fact, the only individuals and organisations who could actually make a formidable stand against societal neurosis would be people and organisations that are totally above suspicion, that is, people who have invested a huge amount of time and effort surviving various quality control procedures. One cannot blame them for thinking, 'Well, I have bent over backwards to live up to all the crazy benchmarks, performance indicators and the like. Why should others have it easier?'

Organisations and individuals who are controllers themselves such as health insurers and patient organisations have a difficult time when policymakers or policy-friendly researchers suggest that they should be watched and monitored as well. You cannot preach transparency and performance standards if you do not practice what you preach.

So what can be done? I believe there are three treatments for societal neurosis to choose from. This may sound reassuring, but these treatments are very much like medical treatments for serious diseases. The first one has severe side effects, much like chemotherapy. The second one requires that politicians, policymakers, and managers commit to a drastic change in behaviour (compare the patient who is suffering from a cardiovascular ailment who has to quit smoking, change his diet drastically, and exercise daily; it can be done, but it is certainly not an easy job). The third one requires the courage and collective action of both professionals and patients. This is probably the most promising treatment, but collective action – as the sociological literature has shown time and again – can be hard to organise, and courage to defy a dominant policy rhetoric and the accompanying instructions to comply is a rare quality in a consensual, corporatist country like the Netherlands. Personally I prefer a combination of the second and the third prescriptions.

The first prescription would be real marketisation instead of bureaucratic marketisation. Let private health insurers try to strike cheaper bargains with hospitals, let them merge with whomever they like, do not ask yourself whether this will interfere with healthy competition, do not worry about insurers who want to select a healthy and youthful clientele, do not discuss the premiums or the differences in premiums for the various categories of patients. In short, if you want to have a market, then have a market. Think about health care the way you think about haircuts. Some people get them regularly, others visit their hairdressers once a year, while others cut their own hair as they see fit. Some have their hair dyed blond, darker, blue, or purple, while others choose perms or an elegant bob. Eccentric individuals want triangles shaved into their heads. Here it is unnecessary to engage in an intricate system of quality control: If people feel their hair has been messed up, they will choose a different hairdresser next time.

Of course, a government cannot abandon health care altogether, there should probably be some emergency care for uninsured people who would otherwise bleed to death in the street, but one could probably stop there and leave the rest up to the people, their insurers, and the health providers.

This prescription of total marketisation might cure societal neurosis, but the treatment may be worse than the disease itself. Health care is not like a haircut; we care whether people are suffering when they could be cured, in a dramatically different way than caring whether people dye their hair a hideous green. Of course, we might organise fund raising events to cough up money to help deserving patients who cannot pay, but we would probably keep having doubts about all the others that we knew nothing about.

The second recipe would consist of the government listening to sensible policy experts who now and then argue that one can definitely have too much of a good thing such as control or accountability. The Dutch scientific council for government policy recently published a report in which they argued that the public service sector was plagued by a huge number of monitoring, checking, and controlling agencies, watching their every move and discouraging all professional initiatives (WRR 2004). The council argued that the government should try to get rid of a lot of these monitoring agencies, learn to trust professionals to do their job on their own and search for different forms of accountability, such as more qualitative reports on what happened and how professionals dealt with it (in fact, very much like Tonkens, cf. her contribution to this volume and Tonkens 2003). The government could also read the chapter by Bovens and 't Hart in an edited volume on public accountability, who argue that too much accountability can be paralysing, time consuming, and frustrating (Bovens & 't Hart 2005). Acting on those insights, however, is terribly difficult. It requires a drastic change of behaviour, which could perhaps only be realised if someone (preferably an economist) could convincingly point out that societal neurosis will in the end stifle economic growth and devour huge amounts of money which might have been spent on real work in health care such as on nurses, nursing home staff, doctors and so on. Paul de Beer's analysis of managerial work (2001) as some kind of non-productive but highly paid activity (not unlike the fake jobs we tend to give to retarded people who cannot hold a proper job because they lack the capacities for that) might be a promising start.

The third prescription is based on the fact that many health care professionals still try to perform their jobs more or less alongside or in disregard of managerial objectives. They care for their patients whether or not this results in a higher score on a balanced score card of performance indicators. Of course this may change in the future. Professionals may become cynical under the weight of an ever larger control structure that forces them to spend ever-increasing amounts of time making plans, writing them down, and evaluating them instead of dealing with patients directly. But at present, although there are probably some professionals who have turned cynical, many have not. And many patients still trust their doctors to help them as best they can; they do not seem eager to engage in a time consuming internet search for the best general practitioner, the best surgeon, or the best hospital (cf. Trappenburg 2005). They visit their family doctor, they know how hard she or he has to work and they can understand their doctor's resistance to increased bureaucratic control.

In 2005, the Dutch general practice doctors decided to go on strike after the government announced its intentions to transfer a substantial sum of money from the incomes of these doctors to that of the health insurers. The rationale behind this was that insurers could then ask them to draw up plans to improve their practices and then reward those who came up with the most promising or original improvements. It was clear that this plan would cut their incomes while placing increased administrative burdens on their backs. A strike might be interpreted as a fight of narrow selfish interests at the cost of patients who were unable to consult their GPs for several days. Dutch GPs are definitely not poor; they earn substantial incomes, so if the strike ended up being perceived as a fight for a few extra euros this could damage their reputations considerably. Despite this, they decided to go on strike and many patients seemed to sympathise with them. In fact, even the media were rather positive about their strike. Unfortunately, in the end, the doctors settled for financial compensation and dropped their other demands, which contributed to the view that they were just in it for the money after all. Still, this strategy of the bonding of professionals and their clients in the primary process may end up being a promising strategy. If professionals engaged in primary care attempt to establish coalitions with their patients (and with those patient organisations who still prefer professionals to insurers, managers, and politicians), if they stick together and simply disregard the tangle of planning and control boards all around them for a while, then common sense may get the upper hand and the protracted process of societal neurosis can ultimately be defeated.

This third treatment might work as a form of shock therapy.

When Ideologies Bounce Back

The Problematic Translation of Post-Multicultural Ideologies and Policies into Professional Practices

Jan Willem Duyvendak and Justus Uitermark

Since the days (1917) that Calvinists and Catholics were allowed to manage their own schools with full funding by the central government, Dutch society has valued the relative autonomy of ethnic and religious groups. The accommodation of immigrant cultures and religions fits with this picture, so it is not surprising that many commentators have labelled the Netherlands a multicultural society (Favell 1998; Joppke 2004; Koopmans & Statham 2000; Koopmans et al. 2005; Soysal 1994; De Zwart 2005). However, developments in recent years have cast doubts upon this image of the Netherlands as a 'multicultural paradise' (Duyvendak et al. 2005; Uitermark 2005). It seems increasingly problematic to label Dutch policies as multicultural, but it would also be misleading to define them as assimilationist. Recent policies seem to combine the two extremes: The push for assimilation is probably stronger in the Netherlands than in many other countries, but at the same time it is clear that policies take into account migrant identities to quite a high degree. In order to solve this paradox, we need to unpack the notion of 'multicultural society'.

In the Dutch debate about the multicultural society, it is striking that little distinction is made between the ethnic-cultural diversity in society as it is in practice, 'multicultural' government policy and multiculturalism as an ideal. Leading critics assume a strong link between the ideal of multiculturalism, the integration policy pursued until recently with respect to migrants, and actual practices at the local level (Scheffer 2000, Schnabel 2000, Van den Brink 2004). On the basis of their observations of unacceptable forms of segregation in cities and institutions, they quickly draw the conclusion that the ideal of cultural diversity is no longer satisfactory and should be replaced by alternative ideals such as 'shared citizenship' and 'national cohesion'.

Historical research (Duyvendak & Rijkschroeff 2004; Fermin 1997; Prins 2000 [2004]; Rijkschroeff, Duyvendak & Pels 2004) has demonstrated that over the last decades, much of the integration policymaking has been driven by pragmatic considerations rather than principles. Moreover, one and the same policy instrument seems to have been applied over time for different reasons, either pragmatic or principle-related (Lucassen & Köbben 1992). To put it another way, policy does not

64

have a one-to-one relationship with ideals; it is based on a variety of motives and justifications as well as principles, and cannot be reduced simply to the implementation of an ideal. An idea that commonly crops up in the public and political debates is that the ideal of a multicultural society permeates all phases of policymaking, including the results, but the literature reveals serious doubts about whether there is a direct relationship between ideas and the actual results of policies (Lipsky 1980; Wilson 1989; Pressman & Wildavsky 1984).

In many studies on multiculturalism, the 'black box' of public administration and how policies are executed remains closed. People assume that there is a close link between the policy pursued and what professionals do in practice. In the Netherlands, policies were multicultural in the sense that they recognised the right of ethnic self-organisation, and due to the religiously 'pillarised' past there was a legal framework that provided rights to minorities (and to other citizens) to follow their own cultural and religious identities. Whether this indeed led to a lot of multicultural practices is an entirely different question – one we want to answer in this chapter on professional practices.

Due to space considerations, however, we cannot investigate the complex relationship between ideals, policies, and practices in detail. What we can do is shed some light on how recent shifts in public debates and the political climate have affected professional practices by briefly discussing two cases.[1] The first concerns the Neighbourhood Alliance, an organisation that shares many of the criticisms that are now often made against multiculturalism. We show that this organisation attempts to translate an ideological critique of multiculturalism into a concrete program. At the same time, we see that there are powerful forces at play on a local level that make it difficult to effectively implement this program. The second case concerns recent reforms of Rotterdam's local right-wing government in which the party of the late Pim Fortuyn is quite hegemonic. This government's mission was to create and implement policies that departed radically from those of the left-wing governments that had ruled Rotterdam for decades. In this case too, we find that the translation of an anti-multicultural ideal into policy practice is not straightforward. Both cases highlight that there are many obstacles that frustrate the translation of ideals into policy and the implementation of policies into practice. These obstacles play their part even when the ideals themselves are hegemonic in the public debate.

The notion that ideals and policies on the one hand and professional practices on the other are closely linked is also a fundamental assumption in the debate on (de) professionalisation: new neo-liberal policies are blamed for limiting the manoeuvring space of professionals (see the many examples in this book). By reconstructing the empirical effects of an ideological shift – and the debate on the integration of ethnic minorities in the Netherlands provides a rather strong example of such a shift – we want to criticise those who suggest a direct relation between policy shifts and professional practices.

A Multicultural Tragedy

It is difficult to overestimate the intensity and scope of the integration debate in the Netherlands. The Dutch have a long and uneasy history with ethnic diversity (Vuijsje 1997). Here we shall only discuss the shifts and developments in the debate since 2000, when Paul Scheffer published his essay on the 'multicultural tragedy'. A quick look at Scheffer's article immediately identifies it as the kind of presentation that became typical of the integration debate. Scheffer uses dramatic and dramaturgical metaphors, saying, for instance, that a multicultural tragedy is unfolding in the big cities in the Netherlands. He also pinpoints the guilty party:

> We are now living with the third generation of immigrants and the problems have only gotten larger. Whether the successful immigrants will play their envisaged role of pioneers remains uncertain, as they usually want to cut loose from their supposed supporters. It is not a sign of open-mindedness to put these observations aside with an easy plea for a multicultural society. All those apologists of diversity do not care what is taking place in the big cities in the Netherlands. (Scheffer 2000)

The heroes in this story are the people who have the courage to break the taboo and talk about the problems of the multicultural society.[2] Scheffer suggested that the Dutch have avoided any serious discussion of the problems associated with migration and the growing ethnic diversity that comes along with it. He warned of the possible formation of an underclass, an ethnic sub-proletariat that lacked both cognitive and economic relations with Dutch society. Arguing that a misplaced sense of political correctness had resulted in the gratuitous embrace of a relativist, multiculturalist ideal, he wanted the Dutch elite to change its attitude. Ethnic minorities should not be encouraged to cultivate their values in their own separate institutions but should instead integrate into society with the full awareness that, in this process, they would lose some of their cultural particularities. Scheffer's argument revolves around the central idea that a diverse and cohesive society can only exist if groups integrate with each other on the basis of widely shared Dutch values. Whereas according to Scheffer policies in the past had been based on the cultivation and separation of ethnic groups (the multiculturalist ideal), he wanted to see the promotion of both ethnic mixing and Dutch values.

This particular discourse on mixing and values was much more widely and strongly held than Scheffer realised when he presented his argument, and this became even more so after his article was published (Prins 2004). Although the debate is extremely complex and wide-ranging, it is not difficult to see that one view is shared by most of the participants: the various ethnic groups had been living too far apart from each other and should now integrate (Entzinger 2003; Ireland 2004; Uitermark & Duyvendak 2004). However, differences arise as soon as the reasons for this situation are discussed. Some blame the intolerance of the Dutch population; others argue that some cultures or religious groups are just not inclined to integrate into any modern society. The first viewpoint is popular among some groups of immigrants (such as the Arabic European League) but it is not very often expressed in public. The latter viewpoint is supported by some of the best-known participants in the debate (like Ayaan Hirsi Ali and Afshin Ellian), but is certainly not hegemonic. The most popular argument is that segregation has been caused by the multicultural ideal of the politically correct elite, an ideal that was not aimed at mixing but at cultivating cultural identities. Overall, we observe a consensus on four points:

1. The government has relied too much and for too long on spokespersons of the various ethnic groups. Since these groups are internally heterogeneous, the legitimacy and usefulness of such spokespersons is by definition questionable;
2. A culture of political correctness among the elite, and in particular integration experts and professionals working with immigrants, has for too long cultivated ethnic differences and made it impossible to discuss the problems of ethnic diversity;
3. Interethnic dialogue is crucial for creating the cognitive and social cohesion that is necessary for collective action and shared responsibility;
4. Migrants in particular, and Dutch citizens in general, can and should develop responsibility for the public good (defined as an ethnically diverse society with basic Dutch values), which is possible if their initiatives are not mothballed by those mentioned under (1) and (2). Showing this responsibility implies that they develop a Dutch identity; double (national) identities are considered an expression of defective loyalty to the host society.

Case 1: The Neighbourhood Alliance

The Neighbourhood Alliance, an Amsterdam-based organisation with local branches, has as its statutory mission to '(further) strengthen liveability in multicultural neighbourhoods and areas'. Its main tool for achieving this goal is creating and supporting 'neighbourhood panels', i. e., 'intercultural resident networks' that develop 'citizen initiatives related to intercultural liveability' (SWA 2004: 21). Such panels are considered important in solving 'a problem in Dutch society: we are living separate lives in isolation from each other, as individuals and as (ethnic) groups' (Ibid: 7). Using the concepts coined by Putnam, the Neighbourhood Alliance argues that there is 'not enough bonding within groups or bridging between groups' (Ibid: 7; compare Putnam 2000). Because of this, the 'public space is at risk of turning into a no-man's land', which will lead to 'a negative spiral' (Ibid.: 7). However, the Neighbourhood Alliance feels that there is an 'immense willingness' to be more involved with each other, on the part of 'both the new and the old Dutch'. The organisation wants to cultivate initiatives that stimulate intercultural communication. 'The use of the word "intercultural" is deliberate. The goal is not a more or less peaceful coexistence of different cultures (known as multiculturalism). Between all residents – including people from different countries – positive social interaction should be created on the basis of a universal Dutch, cosmopolitan identity' (Ibid: 7).

The idea that 'Dutch norms and values' should be promoted through interventions is recent, but it is not unique to the Neighbourhood Alliance. The first Balkenende government (a coalition of the Christian Democratic CDA, the VVD conservative liberals and the LPF, which had become the second largest party even though its leader, Pim Fortuyn, had been assassinated just before the elections) had started a discussion on the nature and significance of social norms in the public sphere and collectively or individually held moral values (see WRR 2003)[3]. The present government, Balkenende II (a coalition of the CDA, the VVD and the social liberals of D66), continues to promote this public discussion. The importance attributed to norms and values has resulted in several policy adjustments and initiatives. For instance, citizenship courses for immigrants no longer contain only practical information and language lessons but also explain to immigrants that the Dutch uphold the separation of Church and state, the acceptance of homosexuality and equality between adults and children of both sexes. Curricula for both elementary and high schools are also being amended to teach pupils the history and importance of Dutch institutions.

The Neighbourhood Alliance – small as it is with an office in Amsterdam where some six professionals work along with dozens of volunteers in urban neighbourhoods – presents itself as an institutional extension of a citizens' movement. Quoting research commissioned by the Neighbourhood Alliance, the organisation suggests that both ethnic Dutch and ethnic minorities are concerned about ethnic segregation and yearn for friendly contacts with neighbours; both ethnic Dutch and ethnic minorities want shared norms and values in their neighbourhoods; more than 75% of the respondents feel that more people should do something and about 50% are conditionally prepared to participate in all kinds of neighbourhood activities (SWA 2004: 16). For the Neighbourhood Alliance, this research raises two questions: Why are there still so many multicultural tensions in neighbourhoods? Why has so little come of these desires and ideals? Their answer is as follows:

WHEN IDEOLOGIES BOUNCE BACK

1. The countless initiatives on a local level operate in isolation. They emerge, blossom... and fade when the momentum is gone. This makes it a huge burden to participate...;
2. The government mothballs spontaneous initiatives because it has stringent requirements regarding representativity and accountability...;
3. The government and welfare professionals have a blind spot for the optimism of residents about intercultural co-operation... They focus on problems and appropriate initiatives and thereby fail to appeal to residents' capacity for self-organisation;
4. There is no 'ideology' for neighbourhood residents... Residents (who want) to contribute to their living environment lack a platform that supports them and protects their interests... (SWA 2004: 16)

This is how the Neighbourhood Alliance defines its position: in opposition to those who frustrate the 'countless' spontaneous initiatives and in support of residents who are prepared to commit to intercultural co-operation. Anti-professionalism and ethnic diversity play a key role here.

The discourse of the Neighbourhood Alliance concerning ethnicity and citizenship is as complex and ambivalent as the integration debate itself. On the one hand, there is a general idea that all citizens should share a common frame of reference and adhere to certain basic values (values which are variously labelled as Dutch, universal, or cosmopolitan – the words are used interchangeably). Cultivating ethnic identities is considered detrimental to social cohesion in disadvantaged neighbourhoods and the organisation regularly deplores the neighbourhood councils for minority organisations, like those in the Transvaal neighbourhood in Amsterdam, where the Neighbourhood Alliance is also active. The Neighbourhood Alliance wants to recruit members to its panel who do not speak on behalf of a specific ethnic group. On the other hand, ethnicity is a constant cause of concern and the growth of ethnic diversity resulting from immigration is considered to be the main problem of disadvantaged neighbourhoods. This makes it very difficult to think of residents simply as inhabitants of a neighbourhood and not also as members of an ethnic group. The solution to this problem, on a discursive level, is to create supra-ethnic identities, to find people who are able to bridge divisions between different ethnic groups and individuals. The discourse of the Neighbourhood Alliance is emblematic of a wider trend towards what we may call post-multicultural policy philosophies (Uitermark et al. 2005). These are regarded as an alternative to the assimilationism promoted in France or Germany. In contrast to assimilationism, post-multicultural policies explicitly take ethnic identities into account. Ethnic identities are constantly evoked and problematised, not neglected or denied.[4] The Neighbourhood Alliance does not seek to give a voice or specific rights to groups, it seeks to negate and negotiate rather than confirm or reproduce group identities.

While dissatisfaction with multicultural policies is now widespread, the Neighbourhood Alliance is one of the few organisations that have translated these criticisms against multiculturalism into a concrete program for social interventions. It should be emphasised that this is quite exceptional in itself. Professional organisations are not often guided by a philosophy but instead operate according to an organisational logic, using professional routines to reach short-term goals. Normally, reorganisations are inspired more by financial considerations or bureaucratic politics than by a reconsideration of policy philosophies or ideologies. The Neighbourhood Alliance is at least a partial exception as it actively draws inspiration from the public debate and tries to turn the debate into practice. It seems to support the idea that there is a direct relation between philosophies and professional practices. But does this policy translate into practice?

When discourse meets practice

We can answer this question by analysing how two different aspects of the Neighbourhood Alliance's discourse play out in the institutional reality of some of the neighbourhoods where it is active: spontaneity versus planning, and ideology versus interest.

Spontaneity versus planning

A feature that is increasingly typical of the contemporary organisations involved in social interventions is the desire to 'help people help themselves', i.e., to undertake one strong intervention in the hope of generating a process of self-organisation. The Neighbourhood Alliance is no exception, since it presents itself as the result of a widely felt desire among residents to participate in the public life of the neighbourhood and to help cultivate positive inter-ethnic relationships through useful and enjoyable activities. This is also the title of a newspaper article on a national meeting organised by the Neighbourhood Alliance for its volunteers: 'The magic of a good neighbourhood lies in spontaneity.' The reality in the neighbourhoods we studied is that citizen initiatives are far from spontaneous and that enduring professional support seems to be a necessary (but not sufficient) condition for achieving sustained activity.

Neighbourhood 8 in Geuzenveld, for which we have the most detailed data, presents a sort of worst-case scenario in the sense that in the end, extended efforts did not result in the establishment of a permanent panel – a stable group of citizens from different ethnic backgrounds that would organise all kinds of activities in the neighbourhood, targeting all residents. Perhaps this case is not typical but it does illustrate the difficulty of organising 'spontaneous' participation. The involvement of the Neighbourhood Alliance in Geuzenveld started in December 2001,

when the organisation contacted some neighbourhood agencies and residents. From December 2001 to April 2002, one community worker of
the Neighbourhood Alliance worked part-time to organise a meeting to
set up the panel. The method was very intensive: she approached people
in the street and went door to door. The community workers of the gov-
ernment-funded Buurtbelangen (Community Interests Committee) supported her in her efforts. Roughly 40 people attended the meeting,
which took place on 8 April 2002.

The first meeting of the panel was held on 23 April and attended by
eight residents, the consultant of the Neighbourhood Alliance and a
community worker from Buurtbelangen. A group of Moroccan girls and
young women formed the core of the panel. At least one consultant from
the Neighbourhood Alliance was always present at the meetings. Other
professionals in the neighbourhood, in particular youth workers, also
attended subsequent meetings. Debated topics included language
courses, a neighbourhood party, the design of (defensible) public space,
a self-help group for Moroccan and Dutch women, a party for girls, the
maintenance of a playground and a Moroccan fashion show. Some of
these activities were carried out successfully but others were not. Here
we are not so concerned with the success or scope of the activities but
only with the input of professionals. Our research shows that this was
very high and that resident participation was low. Professionals were present at all meetings and were sometimes in the majority. Both the Neighbourhood Alliance and the local authorities invested large amounts of
professional energy in order to get the panel started. The professionals
who were involved with the panel, both on the part of the Neighbourhood Alliance and the local authorities, did attempt for a long time to
keep the panel alive, but to no avail. This does not mean that the panel
was entirely unsuccessful – it did organise activities, and some of the
first residents to get involved in the panel have taken up other tasks in
the neighbourhood.

However, all those involved agree that professional input was high
throughout the period but that residents only occasionally developed
minimal levels of self-organisation. The constant investment of professional energy is strongly at variance with idea that, after initial help with
the start-up, residents would be able to self-organise. Anti-professionalism, a core of the Neighbourhoods Alliance's ideology, could not be
translated into practice at all.

Ideology versus interest

Even if it is possible to recruit people into an organisation, actually making sure that they do what they are supposed to do is quite another thing.
This is especially problematic for an organisation that has a strong ideology, like the Neighbourhood Alliance, but does not want to serve any
particular interests or groups. In fact, the organisation wants to bring

together people with very different interests. This creates a situation that is intrinsically difficult to maintain for at least three reasons.

Firstly, any group that claims to serve the general interest is bound to have conflicts with other organisations that have a similar claim and share the same working area. In the case of the Neighbourhood Alliance, these are residents' committees, government agencies, housing corporations, and other organisations. Residents' organisations tend to be dominated by older native Dutch residents. One panel member of Moroccan descent observes that it was a

> missed opportunity. It is a shame since people from so many cultures were involved in the panel... a group of older native Dutch residents felt threatened by the youth. They are still living in the 1960s. They immediately felt they were in conflict with the panel because of the other cultures... They had a 'meetings culture', unlike the minorities who do not know anything about minutes, mailings and so on... They are united in a so-called multicultural residents' group, but in reality it is only native Dutch people who are the ears and eyes of the neighbourhood council.

Conflicts like these often arise as soon as two or more organisations operate on the same turf. The government usually enters as a third party since it has resources, status and influence to allocate. The employees and the director of the Neighbourhood Alliance are normally directly involved in these conflicts and try to protect the interests of the panel. As a consequence, the panel easily becomes a vehicle in a conflict between the Neighbourhood Alliance and a local institutional actor that does not appreciate or acknowledge the role of the panel. Needless to say, these conflicts and competitions for status and resources are not very motivating for members of the panel and tend to have a destabilising effect.

Secondly, co-operation between the Neighbourhood Alliance and local institutional actors may proceed smoothly, as in the case we discussed above, where professionals from the panel and the neighbourhood worked side-by-side. Such a situation may persist for some time but in the long run it is likely that the relationships among different parties will undermine the autonomy of the panel. Since members of the panel ideally share only good qualities (active, open, independent) and lack any clear group membership, they are an asset for any other organisation or group of people who wants to organise activities in the neighbourhood. The girls who formed the core of the panel in Geuzenveld, for example, have now become active in other organisations. There is thus a strong 'pull factor' and there is very little that binds the members of the panel together, since they are selected on the basis of not having strong and durable loyalties.

Thirdly, it must be said that most of the panel members were not directly aware of the ideology of the neighbourhood panel. Sometimes it is explained that the Neighbourhood Alliance does not support activities that do not conform to Dutch standards, like a dance night exclusively for

Moroccan girls (which was then arranged through another organisation). The contact person for the Neighbourhood Alliance is also likely to have some idea of what the organisation stands for. But at a further remove, awareness about the ideology is low. Especially after the initial period of intensive supervision, members are likely to go to other organisations, leave the panel or, if they are not aware of the ideology, support activities that run counter to the principles of the organisation. This was most apparent in The Hague, where members of the Moerwijk neighbourhood panel are presently setting up a special society for Turkish men and another for Turkish women. This goes completely against the philosophy of the Neighbourhood Alliance, but for the members of the panel it is simply one more way to organise activities in the neighbourhood. Since residents who want to get involved in the neighbourhood do not usually support coherent ideologies, they instead pragmatically adjust to whatever circumstances may arise. And since the Neighbourhood Alliance cannot control those circumstances, especially after the period of intense supervision, it is quite likely that the panel ends up merging with other organisations or that its ideology gets watered down.

What can we conclude from this discussion of the Neighbourhood Alliance? The most important observation is simply that there is a world of difference between the national debate and the reality of policymaking in neighbourhoods. The concerns of local actors are not necessarily the same as those expressed in the public sphere. While commentators who participate in the national debate may be concerned about Dutch norms and values or the (lack of) compatibility between Islamic and Western civilisations, most organisations in disadvantaged neighbourhoods simply want to reach their target groups in order to develop and maintain policy interventions. As a consequence, they sometimes end up acting against the very beliefs that are promoted in the public sphere. This is most apparent with the issue of political and administrative organisation along ethnic lines. In the Dutch case, such a constellation is normally not defended on ideological grounds ('each ethnic group should have a seat at the table!') but on pragmatic grounds ('we can only reach immigrants through immigrant organisations'). In a sense, then, examining the exceptional position of the Neighbourhood Alliance helps us understand that most of the time ideology does not find its way into professional practice. When an organisation like the Neighbourhood Alliance explicitly scrutinises professional practices from an ideological viewpoint, it becomes apparent that almost all professional practices fall short of addressing public concerns (as manifested by the public sphere). Interestingly, this is also the case for the Neighbourhood Alliance itself: on the basis of the research we have carried out so far, we conclude that only under very specific conditions (high involvement of headquarters with the panel, high level of professional support, co-operative attitude of other local stakeholders) does its program actually translate somewhat into practice.

Case 2: Rotterdam

Rotterdam is the city in the Netherlands with the most severe urban problems, and it is the only municipality where the populist politician Fortuyn ran for (and won) local elections and where his party became part of the local coalition government. While we can see experiments with post-multiculturalist policies in every major city in the Netherlands, and indeed in Europe, we focus on Rotterdam because this case might show us in an undisguised form the kinds of policies that result when one treats urban ethnic minorities as a new 'dangerous class' (Morris 1994). The discourse on the city by the current local government betrays a strong distrust towards the present residents and a desire to reinstate middle-class norms and values. In line with these new beliefs, numerous policy measures have been implemented in order to make sure that potentially dangerous groups are carefully monitored and disciplined. Zero-tolerance policing is now commonplace and high demands are put on new immigrants to the city; they not only have to learn the Dutch language but are also expected to learn Dutch norms and values. While it was not very difficult to formulate new policy measures, existing professional routines turned out to be remarkably resilient. We illustrate this through a discussion of Rotterdam's social policies, where new ideals slightly altered policies but hardly affected the professional practices at all.

The first example is the so-called 'street etiquette'. The idea for this program was first raised in 1999 by a GroenLinks (Green Left) aldermen who was responding to a growing concern about the manners and behaviour of youths in parts of disadvantaged neighbourhoods. During a city debate, some active residents suggested that the program should be developed for all age groups. The original formulation of the project does not mention ethnicity or crime (Diekstra et al. 2002), it emphasises that street etiquette may reinforce 'liveability'. Citizens needed to become more aware of the consequences of their actions and that the government needed to involve citizens at the neighbourhood level. Street etiquette basically means that residents of a street meet and discuss what they think is 'normal' public behaviour. As a consequence, street etiquette has become a device that is increasingly employed to regulate or test relationships between different groups in disadvantaged neighbourhoods. The current mayor, however, now frames street etiquette as part of a strategy that helps prevent undesirable behaviour – the ambition of creating a positive atmosphere and promoting friendliness seems to have been dropped. At the same time, the agenda is more ambitious since it now appears that street etiquette might even help prevent serious crimes like stabbings:

> The main problems of the city concern safety and filth. The political party programs and the election results show this. These are problems that Rotter-

WHEN IDEOLOGIES BOUNCE BACK

dammers inflict upon each other. Someone is throwing garbage on the street, someone is walking their dog and someone is holding the knife. The most important question in this city is how we deal with each other. Whether we want to take each other into account, whether we agree on rules of communication and conduct. (Opstelten cited in Diekstra et al. 2002: 5)

Thus, the call for a discussion on norms and values is now translated into a call for promoting those kinds of social projects that reduce the levels of insecurity. While the goals here are defined more narrowly and reveal a mistrust of certain groups, the means remain largely the same.

A second example concerns Opzoomeren. This was originally part of the social renewal policy that was formulated in Rotterdam and then transformed into national policy. The basic goal of social renewal was to increase the quality of social relations in disadvantaged neighbourhoods and to promote citizens' initiatives in the voluntary sector. Opzoomeren is perhaps the most famous part of this program: Citizens were mobilised to clean their streets, organise youth and sport activities, and have street barbecues in order to come into contact with each other (Duyvendak & Van der Graaf 2001). Opzoomeren fits in with a more general tendency to empower citizens in order to make them govern themselves and each other. As such, it tends to look for solutions at the community or individual levels rather than the society level. However, at least in its original formulation, it also tried to capitalise on latent citizen qualities: it valued the people living in these neighbourhoods. Opzoomeren, along with a range of other programs, constitutes the cement that needs to bind the different ethnic communities, socio-economic classes and age groups together into a territorial community that has some significance for its members. Thus, while initially the policy was chiefly intended to show some tangible social results for the coalition Christian Democrats, Labour and the Green-Left city government, it is now used in a far more instrumental way for a more specific purpose:

People do not feel safe and do not feel connected to each other and their environment. There is no longer a broad sense of 'us'. There is often distrust among each other and, consequently, in the government. This is indeed the social clash: a contemporary social question. We are confronted with an extraordinary challenge of social integration. (Gemeente Rotterdam 2003: 3)

The new government clearly feels that Opzoomeren can play a pivotal role in meeting this challenge. It has set itself as a target of increasing the number of participating streets from the current 900 to 1,600 in 2006 (that is about half of Rotterdam's streets). It has become part of the new city government's Mensen Maken de Stad (People make the city), a program, which not only encourages residents to undertake activities but also stimulates them to make informal rules as part of street etiquette and to develop an agenda for their own streets: how can the current social situation be improved? This program had been implemented by some 60 to 70 streets at the time of writing (October 2005).

We carried out exploratory research in two of Rotterdam's neighbourhoods (Hoogvliet and Spangen) which revealed that, on the ground, changes were not that significant. In some instances, professionals reluctantly co-operated, but in most cases they considered the new program to be an unwelcome government intrusion. Some professionals even boldly declared that, as far as they were concerned, the city government shouldn't mingle in their business to start with. Most strikingly, was the fact that some of the professionals did not even know there had been a shift in policy. The net result of the policy change is first and foremost an administrative affair, since in many cases, professionals simply continued the same activities as before (Radstaeke 2005).

In conclusion, it is important to note that many policy measures promoting contacts, citizen participation and political inclusion that have already been in place for a long time continue to be supported by the new government. In fact, these programs seem to enjoy even more political support than they did under the previous, social democratic government. In practice, it has been proven very difficult to develop new programs that are a direct response to the call for tougher policies, or even to redesign existing social programs.

Conclusion

Many professionals are concerned that the emergence of anti-professional ideologies constitutes a serious threat to their own practices. For instance, critics of neo-liberalism fear that a belief in the market system undermines their professional discretion. We would suggest that all ideologies are intrinsically difficult to translate into practices.

The difficulty of implementing new philosophies was confirmed by the two cases we examined. In the first, that of the Neighbourhood Alliance, a rather dramatic shift in discourse indeed produced strong but quite unexpected changes in professional practices. Only under very specific conditions (a high level of involvement by the headquarters with the panel, a high level of professional support, a co-operative local stakeholder attitude) was its program somewhat translated into practice. But this comes at a price. While the spontaneity of citizens' initiatives formed a constitutive part of the Neighbourhood Alliance's post-multiculturalist and intrinsically anti-professional philosophy, paradoxically its aims could only be realised in a highly professionalised context (and even then, just partially). The second case, that of Opzoomeren, exhibited an even wider gap between public philosophy and professional practice. Community workers in Rotterdam either resisted, considered the policy change as an administrative burden, or were totally unaware that they were supposed to alter their practices.

In any event, ideology bounced back in both cases. In the first case, residents of neighbourhoods obstructed a direct translation of policies into practices; therefore professionals were forced to adopt the very (dominant) role they abhorred theoretically. Professionals knew what they wanted, but the level of inertia and the complexity of professional practices precluded any direct translation of ideals into reality. In the second case, professionals were either intentionally non-co-operative since they disagreed with the new government, or were unaware of policy shifts – let alone their translation into actual practices in the neighbourhood. This latter form of non-co-operation is quite a surprising result, considering our expectation that the heated public and political debate in Rotterdam would influence professionals, even without direct orders from politicians.

We suspect that what happened (and what did not) in these two cases in a post-multiculturalist Netherlands also applies in other contexts. We obtained interesting insights by looking at the (lack of) professional translation of post-multiculturalist policies into practices, even though the new public philosophy was so overwhelmingly present. If, in this case, policymakers were already experiencing so many hurdles, is it not be plausible to expect an even wider gap between public philosophies and professional practices in situations where public philosophies are more ambivalent or couscious? If so, is this not enough reason to reconsider the general claim in the debate on professionalism that new philosophies and policies are the primary causes of the erosion of professional practices?

Notes

1. The case studies are drawn from Uitermark & Duyvendak 2005a and 2005b, respectively.
2. Fortuyn also presented himself as a rebel who gave politics back to the people by disturbing the political correctness of the governing elites. We can only begin to understand his emergence if we take into account the high profile of the integration issue in the Netherlands and the nature of the political environment (Duyvendak, 2004).
3. Even a superficial discussion on the origins and evolution of the debate on Dutch values and norms would require much more space than is available here. See Duyvendak et al. (2005).
4. The diversity policy is also not an example of old (multiculturalist) wine in new bottles. In contrast to the minority policy previously adopted in the Netherlands, the diversity policy stresses that identities are highly complex and contentious, constantly changing and vary from one individual to another.

PART II

PEOPLE

Safe Neighbourhoods[1]

Sophie Body-Gendrot

Picture this: An elderly police inspector who knows the tricks of his trade. Serial killers, ordinary murderers, drug dealers, rapists, and thieves will no longer walk free as long as he is around to catch them. Accompanied by one or two faithful assistants, he visits crime scenes, interviews witnesses, looks for clues, studies his files, and hunts down the villains until they are safely behind bars. That is, if it is up to him, but usually it isn't. The elderly police inspector whom we know from so many police series on television is very often pestered by the high and mighty, often slightly corrupt politicians, by managers who have never caught a villain in their lives, and by lawyers who see to it that the police abide by all sorts of silly rules. The police inspector is drowned in paper work, has to meet arbitrary targets, has to account for his whereabouts, has to do public relations in the local community and even go to receptions to shake hands with politicians. This is the script of many episodes of many television police series. In this chapter, I intend to show that things are not as simple as that. In fact, I will argue that the politicians, lawyers and managers, and the values they represent can change the culture of professional policing for the better.

All across Europe, the flux of immigrants from developing and formerly colonised countries who are settling with their families in rich European countries, are triggering negative stereotypes in times of macro-mutations and uncertainty. International tensions in the Middle East, concerns about external and internal security, and the blurring of frontiers lead to easy dichotomies of 'us' and 'them' in democracies of opinion, influenced by the media.

In France, formerly thought to be a homogeneous society with now and then invisible flux immigrants irrupting and quietly melting in, the development of more individualistic and culturally diversified society has left national elites and professionals obviously confused, since equal treatment for all does not meet immigrants' special needs. Because former mechanisms of social integration have been eroding throughout the second half of the 20th century and social exclusion has taken new ethnicised forms, current second- and third-generation males often have the feeling they are not fully accepted in the mainstream, and that their trajectories of upward social mobility look dimmer. Having failed at school, and being more or less jobless (with an unemployment rate of 40%, three times higher than that of the general French population) and visibly idle in the public space, collective groups of male youth belonging to 'visible minorities' are frequently perceived and categorised as risks to public safety by large majorities of citizens and the police are required to control their behaviours. In the field, rank-and-file policemen have a large leverage of action that is sometimes labelled as a 'hierarchical inversion' (Salas 2005: 204). Their professional culture leads them to see these youths as 'enemies' even if the latter's potential for violence is of low-intensity. In a mimetic posture, these youths also perceive the police as a rival gang trying to control the public spaces that they have somewhat colonised. They complain of ethnic profiling and of discrimination when they are stopped and frisked.

Similar problems characterise the United States, where the racial issue is more ingrained in the formation of the nation (Dawson 1994). Because the fate of racial minorities has been so singular and their interactions with the police sometimes lethal, until 9/11 immigrants seemed to experience less police abuse in the cities where they settled than historical minorities.

In the Western world, different ways of perceiving and defining situations result in different policies and organisational practices. These perceptions emanate from what could be considered as two contrasting 'models' regarding the justice and fairness for minorities. In France, the essence of the Republican model obeys a logic of equality and not a logic of minorities. The principles of identity and equality are 'founded on the equality of individuals before the law, *whatever their origin, race, religion...* to the exclusion of an institutional recognition of minorities' (HCI 1991: 19; italics in original). Consequently, as institutions do not recognise 'ethnic minorities', it is against the law to include any ethnic or religious characterisation in public statistics.[2] The public debate ignores racism, including institutional racism.

By contrast, since the 1960s, following the civil rights' movement and the rise of Black Power, American institutions have acknowledged the existence of identifiable skin markers, of religious, cultural and national differences, of racism, and of institutional racism experienced by 'visible minorities'. American social policies of affirmative action and judicial decisions in favour of minorities have led to the creation of anti-discriminatory apparatuses based on the rule of law. A major difference with France is that when American local institutions such as the police proceed with reforms, the change is frequently snatched by pressures exerted by organised minority groups acting bottom-up and by legitimised anti-discriminatory organisations which, under favourable circumstances, find political allies in the system of decision-making. By comparison, the French national police are insulated from third-party and mainstream political parties pressures and, as there is no political recognition of the problem, the status quo persists.

Reconciliation of differences may be found in the dilemmas and contradictory injunctions that police forces face in most developed countries. They concern fairness and efficiency. When efficient, the police are accused of ethnic profiling or harassment by those stopped and searched; when fair, they are reproached by conservatives for being 'soft' ('What are the police doing?').

The case of the USA offers a clear illustration of:

1. How and why place matters in a federal and decentralised structure. Two major incidents triggered by the excessive behaviour of local police – the Rodney King and the Amadou Diallo cases – were processed differently by various minority organisations and by the local leadership in Los Angeles and New York and led to different outcomes.

2. The persistence of racial constructions in the attitudes people have, and how they plague minorities and police interactions. Two current issues – racial profiling and police abuse towards minorities – reveal patterns of racial prejudice among police forces (Harris 2003).

3. Justice as it attempts to redress the harm caused to minorities as a category for violating their constitutional rights. When required by judges to stop their discriminatory behaviour after signing a consent decree, police forces in a number of cases have made their files more transparent as a result of litigation. Such bottom-up mobilisations from civil society compel police forces to be more accountable.

The second part shows that in France by contrast:

1. Centralised policies influence the behaviours of national policemen, who are accountable to the government.

2. The official ignoring of race by the French police and a general lack of management of and sensitivity to the issue do not prevent the profiling of immigrant youth, although it cannot be said to what degree the factors of ethnicity, youth and poverty are decisive.

3. Justice's involvement remains marginal on such issues, despite Europe's highlighting of the serious misconduct of the French police. The reluctance of both the government and parliament to document this issue and to improve ethnic diversification in the French police force makes France an anomaly in Europe in terms of institutional accountability.

Concluding remarks argue that transparency and accountability, which are missing in French institutions, are somewhat more easily obtained in the US via strong judicial mechanisms of control, institutional accountability, and decentralised modes of governance. Whenever bottom-up mobilisations defending the improvement of a minorities' treatment by the police are successful, reforms are enforced under judicial or other parties' decisions, but usually only last for a certain number of years – after that, more mobilisations are needed.

In France, timid steps indicate that there is an awareness of the dysfunction of a model based on a logic of equal treatment which is betrayed by institutional practices. Isolated initiatives in some police academies as well as experiments launched by localities to improve police-citizen organisational interactions result in successful partnerships. But as long as society remains indifferent or unwilling to seriously solve the problems giving rise to disorders occurring at its margins, institutions are unlikely to embrace vigorous reforms.

The Police in Problem Neighbourhoods in the US

Policing of US territory is decentralised and comprised of 17,000 local police forces as well as state and county forces.[3] Mayors or commissions appoint police chiefs (in some areas, sheriffs are elected). While, according to the 'broken windows' theory, the police are expected to support citizens' mobilisations in securing their neighbourhoods (Wilson & Kelling 1982), in multicultural cities, the police frequently respond to demands for law and order by frisking the minorities of poor neighbourhoods.

Historically, the relationship between police departments and racial minorities is based on a long series of discrimination, abuse and racial profiling, with the police rarely being sanctioned by their white majorities. According to a 1968 report by Human Rights Watch, the ratio of blacks vs. whites killed by the police in 14 large cities was six to one. In the following decade, minorities mobilised around police brutality issues and racial discrimination, and reforms were observed in a number of police departments. Mayors appointed more minority police officers, and in large cities affirmative action measures boosted the number of minorities in the police forces, before a white-male backlash movement protesting reverse discrimination abated the process. Most large law enforcement agencies have given training in racial and cultural awareness for years. In some departments it is minimal, but in others it serves as an important piece of the puzzle in helping officers understand how race may play a subtle and insidious role in their actions, and how they can become better officers by moving away from profiling (Harris 2003: 171).

Some police departments have particularly brutal reputations. This has been the case of the Los Angeles police department (LAPD), with a record of aggressive law enforcement actions and raids in minority neighbourhoods causing suspicious deaths. The Watts riots in 1965 were triggered by an event that highlighted conflicts between the LAPD and a minority community (Body-Gendrot 1993). In March 1991, an African-American, Rodney King, was brutally kicked out of his car, beaten and badly injured by the LAPD. This time, the episode was recorded by amateur video, and so minority leaders from various organisations had hoped that abusive police officers would be heavily reprimanded by the criminal justice system. Nothing of the kind occurred due to a popular jury in Orange county, where class loyalty towards police officers who tend to live in similar areas was strong. Because there was no justice, there could be no peace for the outraged minority groups. Disorders

and riots then erupted in neighbourhoods around South Central, causing 58 deaths and 2300 injured (mostly among African-Americans) as
well as 5500 arrests (illegal Latinos were deported). This cost the city an
estimated 785 million dollars in damages (Saint-Upéry 1997: V). Minority neighbourhoods paid a heavy price for the riots, while Beverly Hills
and other affluent areas remained intact. A federal investigation commission pointed out LAPD 'racism' and imposed reforms. A Republican
mayor replaced the black mayor of Los Angeles in the following elections. The chief of police was fired, and the new chief promised to
mend the damaged relationship between the LAPD and the minority
community. By 2000, the LAPD included 13.6% African-Americans
(from 9.4% in 1983) and 33.1% Latinos (from 13.6% in 1983). But persis-
tent problems have continued to plague police and minority relationships in Los Angeles since then. Accountability and transparency are basically absent when it comes to the way the police force functions, unless
major turmoil or a scandal turns up in the media and leading voices of
public opinion force the LAPD to perform more fairly and lawfully.

The New York Police Department (NYPD) also experimented with aggressive law enforcement ('zero tolerance') at the demand of New York
Mayor Rudolph Giuliani, a former federal prosecutor. A large-scale experiment that began in the mid 1990s led to numerous stops and
searches of usual suspects as a way of pre-empting and predicting crime.
Race emerged as part of the profile. In minority communities, residents
felt that the NYPD's tactics were unfair and racially motivated. In this
context, one would expect that a similar case of police abuse against an
African immigrant – Amadou Diallo, killed by mistake after 41 bullets
were shot at him by a street crime police unit in February 1999 – would
have generated massive riots protesting biased treatment. Why this did
not occur is intriguing. One of several explanations concerns the leadership exerted by black organisations' leaders and local authorities: both
managed to contain disorders in the city and converted them into actions of civil disobedience. The tradition of progressive politics that characterises New York thus led more than 2000 residents of all races, ages,
and social status to demonstrate on the streets demanding police reforms. The NYPD was subjected to state and federal investigations, the
policemen involved in the shooting were sanctioned, ethical codes were
reinforced, street crime units dismantled, and more ethnic and racial
recruiting took place. Popular mobilisations combined with the Federal
Department of Justice intervention were determinant factors in the enforcement of reforms. Former incidents of NYPD police brutality had
already been exposed, but it was their cumulative effect and the mayor's
vulnerability at that time that forced the institution to bend to new forms
of accountability.

The 150-year history of the NYPD, as analysed by Johnson (2003),
reveals cycles of approximately ten years between reforms against police
brutality. For instance, clubbing was a routine practice of patrolmen in

the 19th century, bludgeoning citizens with nightsticks or blackjacks. After the first state committee, the Lexow Commission, exposed police corruption and misconduct in 1894, a police reformer, Theodore Roosevelt, was nominated and he implemented stricter disciplinary practices. The following period, 1900-1911, reveals a typical feature of New York, the capacity of its racial and ethnic groups to organise, which corroborates the ideas developed by Katznelson in 'City Trenches' (1981) relative to a dual mode of organization: a working class unitary one in the factories and an ethnic and racial one at the neighbourhood level. Typically, police issues reveal that new immigrants and racial minorities are subjected to hostility from settled white populations when they cluster in specific neighbourhoods. The level of brutality or protection they receive marks their changing positions on the scale of power. It was only after 1905 that a patrolman was successfully found guilty of the murder of an African-American, and in 1911 the first black officer was hired by the NYPD. The progressive era showed that stopping police brutality and reducing the number of arrests could become a political priority. But reformers become vulnerable when crime rises, which was the case during the early 1900s. Although the goal was praiseworthy and prominent judges sided with him, New York Mayor Gaynor had to abandon his efforts. It was only in 1931 that the 11th clause of the Wickersham Commission report condemned lawlessness in law enforcement, especially the 'third degree' applied to indigent, non-influential suspects and minorities as a particular discipline meant to force them to conform to the law without consent. Again, efforts to create a civilian review board were marred by police interest groups, claiming as usual that this would tie the hands of police officers while giving more power to the criminals. A cyclical pattern emerged that expressed itself as the swing of a pendulum between repression and reforms. Citizens, the judicial system, city authorities, federal initiatives, or even the global context generates these processes. For instance, the Vietnam War and 9/11 have both had an impact on NYPD practices and priorities.

A more recent case has drawn attention to local police forces. Racial profiling is defined as a highly discretionary police tactic that activates the police suspicion of minorities and turning profiles into police investigations (Harris 2003). The police justify these actions as an effective crime-fighting tool. But this selective orientation goes against the Constitution, which offers equal protection to all and protects citizens from unreasonable searches and seizures. Minorities who have been stopped and frisked based on profiling often know that they have been singled out because of 'race-making situations' (Fagan 2002: 150 n. 47). Not only does this profiling hurt them emotionally, but also these situations can escalate into violent encounters, a situation similar to that experienced in France's problem areas. Minority residents thus feel that they share a linked fate of submission to police relations of domination, and that it is in their interest to respond collectively.

In the case of racial profiling along New Jersey Turnpike, minority drivers complained about being stopped in far greater numbers to their presence on the road to the point that the highest court had to restrict the use of consent searches in New Jersey in 2002. They found that these searches played a major role in racial profiling. Blacks comprised 13.6% of road users but 73% of those being stopped. Two troopers involved in the shooting of four young unarmed black athletes after they were pulled over freely admitted that they had resorted to racial profiling. They added that they had been trained to do so (Harris 2003: 55, 240). The consent decree signed subsequently between the state police and the US Department of Justice not only prohibited racial profiling in most circumstances except specific ones, it requested troopers to base every consent search on the written consent of the driver. A dozen other states have followed suit.[4]

In the above cases, the institutions have since learned their lessons and trained their forces better. Accountability in the American tradition has served here to reveal brutal police practices, which are less and less tolerated by better-organised minorities and which force institutions to reform themselves. But it goes without saying that minorities are not so well organized in numerous cities and that place matters. The behaviour of the police in New Orleans after the hurricane of 2005 is an example. Even in large cities where minorities act as watchdogs on police actions, the struggle has to be continuous due to the cycles between reform and brutality already described. The context of the time such as the aftermath of 9/11 also has an impact, jeopardizing already gained civil rights' victories. However, even if it is fragile, the notion of institutional accountability is ingrained in the U.S. This is not the case of France, where institutions and their elites are almost never sanctioned and where accountability is unknown due to historical circumstances. The State made the nation, patiently under the monarchy, then under the Republic. The French tradition is to rely less on justice and more on internal inspection corps (some dating back to the monarchy) to sanction delinquent police officers.

The Police in Problem Neighbourhoods in France

How different is the French posture from that of the American? To begin with, France has a national police force, accountable to a centralised Ministry of Interior, or in the case of gendarmes, to the Ministry of Armies, and not to the citizens of France. Top-down policies regarding police missions have changed a lot over the last years, and policemen complain about constant reforms and the instrumentalisation of their work by the political elites for electoral gains. In the 1980s, efforts were made to create a form of community policing, establishing more trust between the police and citizens. Policemen were to be partners in the elaboration of crime prevention schemes and to act moderately in terms of repression. (The police were, however, seen walking the beat less often than they were seen patrolling problem areas by car, and they saw their role more as conveying the grievances of crime victims to the justice system than developing better relations with multicultural populations.) Although the Council of Europe has since 1994 required that the police develop a more accurate, respectful and sensitive vision of various ethnic and racial groups (Conseil de l'Europe 1994: 15, 19) and in spite of the injunction of the French Ministry of Interior in 1999 that the police should better reflect the populations they serve, the institution has proven resistant to performing social missions instead of mere order maintenance. It has been equally reluctant to open its ranks to second- and third-generation immigrants, and it has chosen to assign this task to private security agencies and municipal local forces.

In the mid-1990s, when fear of crime was a serious French middle-class concern, more repression and risk management methods were introduced in police departments by the ruling Left government, a trend which culminated in 2002, during a time when crime was the major concern of the French. Since then, a new policy focussed on zero tolerance for delinquents has given more leverage to policemen and prosecutors as it is done in the U.S. Stricter measures for the judicial treatment of youths at risk were elaborated (Body-Gendrot 2005), and a new punitive populism was said to have been politically stimulated by a Minister of Interior with Presidential ambitions (elections are to take place in 2007).

French policemen are often beholden to contradictory injunctions from their superiors: On the one hand, they are expected to control and instil social discipline among the marginalised, idle, and visible male youths whose very profile is perceived as a risk and who are thus under control of different police forces constantly patrolling their neighbourhoods. Police are graded on the number of stops and searches that they carry out. On the other hand, they are also required not to inflame the neighbourhoods where they operate for fear of hostile media coverage, and are asked to maintain social peace – a rather difficult task in areas largely deserted by other social institutions. This posture partly explains why disorders in November 2005 after two purportedly fleeing the police were accidently electrocuted lasted three weeks. The police showed restraint in many cases, preferring insurances to pay for the 8 700 torched cars, 255 schools, 233 public buildings, 51 post offices vandalized or burnt in 300 neighborhoods rather than hurting lethally some youth. As a consequence, only one death was reported (for the other death, it is unclear).

A second difference between the French and American police involves the official ignoring of race, a term that cannot be easily translated from one country to another. Histories and structures vary, semantic spaces and social traditions differ. Race is a construction marking boundaries.

Few statistical tools allow French researchers to document racist attacks, cases of ethnic discriminations and ethnic profiling. How many second- or third-generation French citizens have been stopped and searched? How many are imprisoned? Do these questions matter? The fact that more than half of the prison population in the US is African-American male allows anti-discrimination organisations to build their cases hoping that under favourable political and economic circumstances at the states' level, they will push the repressive pendulum back in favour of preventative measures. But in France, such a case cannot even be made.[5]

That some policemen are racists and act accordingly is not acknowledged as such by the police institution, which on the whole is not accountable to citizens. However, this institutional ignoring of race takes place in a context marked by the phenomenon the ethnicisation of social relations. Using the rhetoric of the extreme right, the transformation of former 'dangerous classes' (the working class) during the first half of the 20th century (self-labelled Apaches, zulus or black jackets) into males of immigrant origin concentrated in large public housing projects clearly shows that similar processes of externalization continue to operate under different forms. From a law-and-order point of view, 'otherness' remains situated at the economic and spatial margins and the usual suspects are found in the same decaying urban areas. Policemen reflect the stereotypes of mainstream society, a society in which 40% of the population claims "understanding" for extreme right, racist and xenophobic ideas. 'Judging individuals according to their supposed ethnic characteristics occurs during the professional socialisation of the police. Racist representations have an instrumental function in order to differentiate individuals' (Zauberman & Levy 2003). French policemen deny racial profiling but admit that due to the logics of context, some policemen may overreact in situations of stress, when outnumbered.

The question of space is an important issue here. In marginalised neighbourhoods, youth's spatial identities are established in and through relations of domination and subordination. Distinctions do not emanate from essentialised identities as they do in the US, but from territorial coalitions formed in early youth (Body-Gendrot 2002). Religious, racial and ethnic differences are thus perceived by French and immigrant youth as secondary to an identity of belonging to the collective space of the banlieues. Space as well as respect are important to them because they own so little. The very fact that the youths, many of them of Arab-Muslim origin, want to control and almost privatize this collective space is what troubles the police. Youths' conception of the ownership of space (no-go areas) indeed contradicts the generally shared vision of public space and is perceived as 'uncivil' and threatening.

As for policemen, the interviews we carried out during our two-year investigation display a large range of opinions, attitudes, and judgements (Body-Gendrot & De Wenden 2003). Among rank-and-file policemen, some discard all immigrant residents as troublemakers, drug users, and fundamentalists, while some who reluctantly avow having racist biases claim they would never engage in discriminatory behaviour (it was impossible to find any policeman who had been sanctioned to talk or to find colleagues of such a policeman who would speak out). Still, many admitted that, after being subjected to continuous provocations by a number of well-organised troublemakers, now and then they 'blow a fuse' and overreact. On the whole, most of them, already serious family men, noted that in the deprived neighbourhoods they felt despised by the population who spit on them, stone their cars, insult them – all this plus a general indifference from mainstream society, except when disorders last over three weeks and when threats of contagion are feared as was the case in November 2005. There is no relationship between the officers and the districts in which they work. They are recruited from throughout the country and assigned according to needs; many end up in a city they don't know very well, and they spend the better part of their careers attempting to return to their own region through a series of transfers (Zauberman & Levy 2003). Policemen often experience fear, either of being injured or cause an injury. In our interviews, they all complained about a lack of training, contradictory missions, and a lack of support from their superiors.

The third major difference between French and American police departments concerns the weak position of the French department of justice to redress institutional discrimination. As is the case in numerous countries and in the US as well, judges are reluctant to condemn policemen for their misbehaviour. In 1995, only 21 out of 253 complaints led to the convictions of police officers, and in 1996 12 out of 166 (Jobard 2002). If internal sanctions do occur (between 250 and 350 each year), the public is not informed, which confirms the lack of transparency. In 2002, only 2% of French policemen were sanctioned by police inspectors, while police violence has shown a 6% increase over the past few years (and even more than 6% of registered violence in 2003), according to official reports of the Inspection Generale des Services (IGS).[6]

A culture of denial thus characterises the French police department, and its standard line of defence is that police abuse is an exception. Moreover, in those cases where abuse cannot be ignored, the public service system shields policemen from the legal sanctions that apply to ordinary citizens, again a pattern also observed in the US. An episode documented in detail by French researcher Fabien Jobard illustrates these points (2002: 3). It opposed the European Committee for the Prevention of Torture (CPT)[7] created by the European Court of Human Rights (ECHHR) and France on the use of torture by the French police, for which they were convicted twice – in 1999 (Selmouni case) and in 2002 (Mouisel case).

The racist dimension of urban disturbances is rarely acknowledged and is never used as evidence in the response of state authorities to the CPT accusation. After seven visits to France, the commission pointed to 'a non-negligible risk of being mistreated' at police stations. The European conviction of the French police, who are already perceived as brutal and cynical, came as no surprise to observers. The surprise came from elsewhere. The government mobilised to defend its police force, making efforts to require proof of abuse and making a distinction between well-grounded accusations and slanderous charges. The government asserted that the 'guarantees surrounding the use of force by the police in France and the code of ethics of the National Police were enough to reduce the risk of mistreatment'. The commission emphasised the fact that it was a small sample of allegations of violence that was monitored by disciplinary and control commissions within the police. In other words, the government played down the charge: police transgressions were rare and allegations were not considered valid evidence. It is unusual for French judges to side with vulnerable categories against policemen, anyway. Judges have much difficulty leading inquiries involving the police and the obtaining complete police files and this is not unique to France, it also happens in the US. The cases frequently end up being closed for lack of evidence, even more so on appeal.

Inquiries involving the police meet numerous obstacles, cases drag on forever due to police reluctance to forward documents to judges, and cases are frequently closed for lack of evidence. Policemen are cynical about the impunity their status grants them. Sometimes judges get tired of having to face the same policemen who are repeatedly charges of rebellion, and choose to dismiss the cases on the spot.

Fabien Jobard and Marta Zimolag (2006) have studied the decisions of a French district court involving cases against policemen holding public authority between 1965 and 2003.[8] The issue was whether ethnic discrimination had occurred, based on the ethnicities of individuals arrested and convicted because of their contempt towards a policeman. Contempt in France is punishable by a six-month prison term and a 7,500 euros fine. It consists of 'any words, gestures or threats... addressed to persons in charge of a public service mission... liable to undermine their dignity or the respect owed to the office they hold' (art. 433-5 of the Criminal Code). Obstruction is defined as 'displaying violent resistance to a person holding public authority' (art. 433-6 of the Criminal Code). It receives the same punishment as contempt. The third offence is assaulting an officer, which is always a misdemeanour.[9] Over 1,500 cases were judged between 1965 and 2003 in one specific district court, located in the Paris periphery. The period reveals an increase in cases of outrage and rebellion in that court, which are not just the result of an increase in population. The number of actual delinquents rose only slightly. The explanation can also not be the growing level of 'roughness' observed in social relations in French urban life since the mid-1980s. The reason can mostly be attributed to changes in the criminal justice system that has encouraged the police to classify an entire series of acts as misdemeanours, requiring that the person be taken in and placed in custody. The main correlation between these cases and violent-offence measures, then, is that the new micro-sociological infrastructure of interactions (in terms of duration and intensity) between offenders and the police has been the result of changes in the criminal legal provisions in France. This in-depth reform is noteworthy and is bound to have an impact on the rioters arrested during the autumn disorders of 2005.

Between 1960 and 1980, few cases were taken to court, and the police only processed the cases they felt were the most serious. Today, quite the opposite is occurring: The police now send all their cases to court. What is even more noteworthy is that police officers tend to add the charge of obstruction to their contempt cases to make sure that the offenders will be prosecuted – as proof of their discretionary powers. Another explanation assumes that the public prosecutor has taken the initiative and asked the police to show preference for obstruction cases, since they are deemed to be more 'serious' than mere contempt charges, despite the fact that they receive equal sentencing.

What is interesting in this study concerns the profiles of the offenders. A very large proportion of the youthful defendants are North African and strikingly young (for the period in question, 50% are under 22 and 25% under 18). The types of offences prosecuted vary according to the various groups. North Africans are prosecuted less often for contempt alone and more often for assaulting a police officer or for contempt plus obstruction than defendants in 'other' categories. 24% of the North Africans judged as repeat offenders in real-time case processing are given unsuspended sentences versus 7% of those in other categories of offenders.

It should also be noted that unemployment is highest among youths of North African origin. Given the role played by social discrimination, the judicial system automatically sanctions those not offering guarantees of social conformity. Although generalisations cannot be drawn from a single district court, Jobard and Zimolag (forthcoming) conclude that 'court decisions pitilessly echo and multiply the singularities of a population which differs both in its origins and in its relations with the criminal justice system in that it is more wont than any other group to be in contact with the judicial system'.

The same anomaly of unsanctioned ethnic discrimination is found among the administrative review boards and various other commissions handling infringements by security or police officers. Whereas in other countries (Canada, the US, the UK), citizens' grievances relative to police misbehaviour are recorded, in France citizens can only summon the National Commission on Ethics via a member of parliament. In the first year of operation of that Commission (2001), there were only 13 court cases against the police, by the second year this number was 100. While the commission makes no judgements or decisions, it does have investigative and interviewing powers and does issue recommendations, thus giving visibility to cases of misconduct. However, a strategy of the current government (in 2005) is to systematically deprive the commission of the most elementary material resources to conduct its investigations.

Conclusion

In both the US and France, the lack of appropriate training and supervision of rookies is noticeable. Low-status policemen end up dealing with low-status 'clients' with a large level of personal discretion – called an 'inversion hierarchy' by Salas (2005). It may be assumed that one way these rank-and-file policemen mark their distinction is to resort to a 'confined violence', which is made possible by its covert nature and by the fact that it occurs in grey areas where there are often no witnesses. This is especially true in France, where few citizens in problem neighbourhoods are ready to come forward to the courts, due to the fact that these 'usual suspects' find it impossible to file legal complaints as well as to the absence of third parties (such as public prosecutors) and anti-discriminatory organisations to monitor and control the abuse. In other words, both the delinquent policemen and the delinquent youths are the leftovers of indifferent mainstream societies, political representations, and institutions that choose to ignore what is going on at their margins (Ocqueteau 2002: 210). Rank-and-file policemen often have the feeling that they are enforcing the 'dirty work' of control, surveillance, and arrests in marginalized urban areas because other integrative institutions (family, educational, social, occupational) have neglected their missions. A proof of this neglect was revealed not only by the three weeks of disturbances in November 2005 but by the astounding silence of the state, months after they took place. The heart of the matter is that the state does not know what to do: it only acts on the long-term, while the media impose more and more short-term visions and it only knows how to act technocratically and mechanically while local à la carte solutions would be appropriate.

In the US, the fact that police abuse and its dysfunctions are now monitored as discussed earlier does not mean that the brutal practices are coming to an end. As long as they are not caught, some police officers may still be tempted to exert their monopoly of violence in harmful ways, until bottom-up initiatives supported by organised minority leaderships, the media and/or political reformers call for justice that imposes new regulations. Most of these regulations are only temporary, as the aforementioned case in New York demonstrates. This does not apply to the entire nation, however, as law and order remains the most important local issue. The US appears to have a toolkit with various modes of accountability and transparency emanating from its 17,000 police forces.

In France, the fact that police are being less brutal with citizens than in the past can be somewhat measured by the decreasing numbers of civilians killed by police officers (although police brutality in general

continues to rise), thus supporting the observation that European societies are in general less prone to violence than American society. Self-de-
fence is not legitimate. But the impunity with which some policemen
interact with ethnic and racial minorities damages French democratic
ideals. Recently, during the disorders, a resident formulated his grie-
vance as such: local policemen know the bad apples, they know the drug
dealers and the thugs as we do. But the swat police (CRS) treat us all
without distinction, with the same utter lack of respect. A study conducted by Wieviorka and his team, and subsequently corroborated by
numerous other researchers, concludes that for the French police, a pervasive racist discourse is a reality and constitutes an actual norm, which
is extremely difficult to escape, not to speak of opposing if you are a
rank-and-file officer (1992: 261). That functional racism is part of police
culture and has a reactive character is a remark that also applies to the
American situation. But the French system in particular lacks the initial
and on-going training of policemen, and the lack of accountability to
anyone other than headquarters (Zauberman & Levy 2003). The accountability to the citizenry of France remains an unfamiliar concept
that is seldom discussed. This is one of the reasons why community
policing did not last long and why evaluations of public policies remain
so uncommon.

The entire elite culture that was inherited from the monarchy has enough resources to resist demands for democratisation, and in the case of
the police, very strong police unions buttress the institution, which has
isolated it from third-party pressures.[10] Now and then, the media evoke
police reforms that have taken place abroad, but mostly as something
exotic. A sort of cultural fatalism[11] prevails, actively supported by self-
interested elite groups, echoing the 'nothing works' lament that characterised the American justice system back in 1996.

Nevertheless, in a few police academies, such as the one in Marseilles,
reforms concerning more transparency have taken place. The syllabus
has been modified and it now includes training courses focussed on police interactions with residents. The location of the police academy in a
problem area facilitates a partnership with local community organisations eager to improve the quality of public services and to introduce
future policemen into residents' perceptions about conflictual issues.
These innovations remain the exception, however. It is as if the Minister
of the Interior is afraid of losing control if policemen are allowed to express their fears and resentments too openly. Other experiments have
been initiated by local professionals involved in youth services who often
reach out to policemen and organise forums between obvious conten-
ders. They are noteworthy but remain isolated exceptions.

Most societies offer few incentives to convince experienced educators,
police officers, and judges to accept assignments in the troubled areas in
order to give these residents the same chances as the rest of society. It is
easier to ignore and suppress the violence at the margins. This political

and social short-sightedness may explain why governments so frequently bow to police authorities and their unions when these tend to minimise or deny any wrongdoing. This phenomenon is even more pronounced in a centralised country like France, which has a national police force.

Notes

1. This article is based on a two-year seminary conducted with Catherine de Wenden under the auspices of the Group for Study and Struggle Against Discrimination in France (Geld) in 2000-2002 and on field work on police issues in sensitive neighbourhoods carried out in both France and the United States between 1997 and 2004.

2. After France suffered from terrorist attacks, the Commission monitoring the processing of personal data (CNIL) agreed that 'objective, unalterable distinguishing physical marks' could be included in the police database. This concession was done despite loud protests by civil rights advocates as well as by right-wing conservatives. But later on, when police tried to use a suspects' skin colour after their participation in collective urban violence, the Socialist Minister of Interior stated that it was against 'the values of the Republic' to do so and the matter was not pursued (Le Monde, July 8 and 11, 1997; Zauberman & Levy 2002).

3. There is a complex division between them and an overlapping of authorities, although in special cases, the FBI may legally take over a local police force's fields of intervention. For a description of the fragmentation of police forces in a city like New York, cf. E. Conlon 2004: 12.

4. In 2000, investigations led by Attorney General White and New York State Prosecutor Spitzer showed that ethnic profiling was pervasive. Half the African-Americans (25% of the population) were stopped and searched, which was more than Latinos (one-third had stopped and searched) and whites (13%). In the State of New York, one and a half million dollars were spent to address the situation, creating files on police activities that were being monitored for ethnicity and race (like in the UK).

5. A study indicates that 43% of those under judicial supervision are the offspring of two foreign-born parents (Choquet 2000). Khosrokhavar estimates that in the 18 to 24-year-old group, those with a North African father are 9.27 times more likely to be arrested than those whose father was born in France (2004: 280). That the judicial system convicts immigrant children more often (due to poverty, racism, multiple acts of delinquency) is not surprising.

6. Most of the sanctions are summons. Fewer than 200 policemen were fired in 1999 (Jobard 2006).

7. Article 3 of the European Convention for the Protection of Human Rights passed in 1950: 'No one may be subjected to torture or to inhuman or degrading punishment or treatment'. The CPT is an independent organisation that is allowed to visit prisons, police stations, psychiatric institutions, etc. at any time and without warning if there is suspicion of mistreatment.

8. This section draws on a chapter to be published in Comparative Perspectives on Legitimacy and the Criminal Justice System, Sampson et al. (eds.), New York: Russell Sage (forthcoming).

9. The English translation of article 111-1 of the French Penal Code states that criminal offences are categorised according to their seriousness as felonies, misdemeanours or petty offences. Felonies are serious crimes and are judged by popular juries, misdemeanours are offences judged by penal courts, and petty offences calling for fines are judged by police courts.

10. On November 14 2005, a national police union called on its members in the Parisian banlieues to engage in a work slow down in protest of sanctions ordered by the Minister of Interior on few officers involved in the beating of a few youth during the disorders.

11. To echo a Minister from the French Fourth Republic, "there is no serious problem that a lack of action will not solve".

When Diversity Matters[1]

Marleen van der Haar

> Lately I have had a lot of Turkish clients, a lot of Turkish women... and that is strenuous in a completely different way than working with Dutch women. There is a very big difference indeed... I think because of culture... there are many stress complaints and also little self-reflection, at least with the women I have seen up till now.
> (Interview with social worker, 7 October 2003)

Introduction

Human service organisations are confronted with a culturally plural clientele. This study intends to unravel the everyday practices of social workers in dealing with cultural diversity. Assuming diversity has an impact on both the general repertoire and the everyday work of professionals, the question of this chapter is: How do professionals deal with diversity? I will focus mainly on what social workers experience in the providing of social services to a culturally diversified clientele: How do social workers talk about cultural diversity and how do they relate these issues to their professional attitude and competence in their own words?

Following Hall, Sarangi and Slembrouck (1997; 1999), I will describe the professional activity of social workers as a discourse practice. Accordingly, I assume that social work practices do relate to 'general' or 'societal' discourses (Foucault in Blommaert & Bulcaen 2000) provided by society at large, by the profession or by the organisation at hand. Furthermore, I assume that their everyday interactions on the work floor are influenced by these general discourses, however much these local interactions should also be seen as local discourses in the sense of local 'processes of mutual sense-making' on their own behalf.[2] Accordingly, I intend to demonstrate how in the interview accounts perceptions on 'culture' are, at least partly, framed by the focus on individualisation and empowerment that appears to dominate the current social work discourse.

Dealing with Migrants in the Social Sector

In the Netherlands, roughly half a million people (about 3% of the Dutch population) contact the social services office annually (VWS 2004). Of those contacting a social worker, the percentage of clients with a country of origin other than the Netherlands fluctuated from 16% in 2000 to

97

23% in 2002 (NIVEL 2004: 134). These data largely correspond with those of the studied organisation.[3]

Nevertheless, the starting point of this chapter lays not so much in a rapid or sudden increase in the number of migrant clients with appointments with Dutch social workers. This chapter is motivated by the fact that dealing with immigrants[4] in Dutch professional settings is generally perceived as difficult and is often problematised by means of 'culture'. Referring primarily to the mental health care sector in the Netherlands, Van Dijk and Van Dongen (2000) declare that nowadays 'culture' is frequently perceived as the main reason and explanation for the labelling of immigrant clients as a 'problematic group'. In the case of social work, De Vries (2000: 109) points to a similar tendency of reducing all problems to single aspects, like cultural differences and traumas (in the case of refugees).

Obviously, culture can be used as an instrument to mark boundaries between the imagined yet experienced 'us' and 'them'. An accent on differences in an interaction with 'cultural others' can often be perceived, as knowing one belongs to something that is not part of the 'other' creates a feeling of order and safety. Bulcaen and Blommaert show that social work practitioners in Belgian urban shelters for migrant women have incorporated rather fixed black-and-white schemes 'that identify "cultures" and put them in opposition to each other' into their professional repertoire, pre-structuring the actual path of assistance (1999: 7). They also find that professionals often use culture both as a descriptive category (used to describe the client's context) and as an explanatory category (used as an all-determining factor and explanation of the client's problem). A Finnish study (Anis 2005) of social work encounters with immigrant families also reveals problems in terms of culture. This study provides a more nuanced insight into the complexities of everyday practice by identifying three ways of using 'culture' as a resource: culture is used to explain the 'normal' as opposed to the 'otherness' presented by migrant clients, as an indication and an explanation of the 'difficulty' one encounters, and as a methodological tool in creating dialogue (Anis 2005).

Simultaneously, in society at large – at least in most European countries – the multicultural society is a contested issue in political and public debate. Again, the concept of culture plays a significant role. To illustrate, in her book *Generous Betrayal* Wikan (2002) discusses the sometimes unbearable consequences of a culturalist perspective and shows how in everyday life excessive respect for 'their culture' blinded the Norwegian government (here she also refers to social workers and other professionals in human services) even to the point of 'betraying' help-seeking Norwegian citizens with immigrant backgrounds, because of a widespread conviction that the problems of immigrants are best solved 'within their own group'. She emphasises the issue of individual and collective identity: 'Whereas Norwegians generally regard other Norwegians as individuals with a different character and ability and will to think for themselves, immigrants are largely perceived as products of culture' (Wikan 2002: 81). Wikan points out a double standard, which means that 'culture' is applied to immigrants and not to 'ourselves' (in this case Norwegians). She argues that culture has become a holy cow that breeds impotence, intolerance and irresponsibility (Wikan 2002: 83). Benhabib (2002) in her book *The Claims of Culture* also speaks of the use and abuse of culture.

Besides Wikan and Benhabib's criticisms, Struijs and Brinkman, in their book *Clashing Values* (original title Botsende Waarden) that offers guidelines for the Dutch social sector on ethical issues in multi-ethnic client situations, point out the fact that culture should first and foremost be treated as a necessary 'context of choice' for the individual, instead of it being understood as a fixed identity that evidently belongs to and fits all of its 'members'. That is to say, this perspective takes culture as heterogeneous and emphasises that it provides individuals with a range of options out of which they can construct their own lives (Ibid).

Additionally Baumann's (1999) idea of a dual discursiveness of the positions of essentialism and constructivism is a central stance. Hereby one acknowledges that, in everyday life, people also make use of essentialism and reification while making sense of the world around them. That is, meanings are continuously constructed and reconstructed, and therefore can also be produced as static and fixed within a situated process of sense-making – or better yet, as Gastelaars and Vermeulen argue, 'their reification is a fact insofar as it is continuously produced locally' (2000: 10).

Research Material

This chapter presents the results of an ethnographic study in the social work department of a social services organisation in a medium-sized Dutch city. The social work department provides first-line psychosocial help and employs about thirty social workers, including two trainees. The fieldwork consisted of a three-month period of full-time research on location in 2003. Some additional research was conducted in 2004.

The main research material consists of interviews with social workers and observations of interactions between the professionals and their clients, both native and migrant, and observations of meetings between social workers (like team and inter-vision meetings), and between social workers and other professionals. The material additionally includes documents, client files and interviews with management and other significant organisational members.

The interview material on which this chapter is based consists of semi-structured, in-depth interviews with 16 social workers.[5] Eleven interviewees were female, five male (this corresponds roughly with the composition of the social work team). The age of the social workers varied between 23 and 55 (with an average age of 37). The interviewees also varied in work experience in the organisation (from about a year to over 24). Three interviewees could be categorised as having non-Western immigrant backgrounds (including one trainee), with the rest of the social workers having an ethnically Dutch background.

A Diverse Clientele: From a Categorical to an Integral Approach

More than 20 years ago, the Dutch government introduced a policy to incorporate specialised organisations for immigrants into general social services agencies (Goewie 1986; Hueting & Neij 1991: 193). The policy aimed particularly at a categorical approach within general human service organisations. This means that social services organisations were expected to appoint a specific employee in order to develop programs for their migrant clients (Goewie 1986: 13). Accordingly, the organisation studied employed professionals who specialised in social work for specific immigrant groups like Turks, Antilleans and Surinamese.

Currently, the organisation's policy towards clients is based on an integral approach, which in Dutch social-work jargon implies that all clients are approached in a similar manner and that professional categorical treatment was no longer permitted; every single professional is expected to be able to help every single client according to his or her individual needs. This new policy put an end to the organisation's offer of categorical assistance to the aforementioned migrant groups as well as to the numerous mobile-home dwellers who also live in that region.

Nevertheless, some categorical assistance continues to exist. The organisation still benefits from the specialisations of some of its social workers (for example working with Turkish or Antillean clients, or working with client categories like families or specific groups). The main change is that separate departments or individual social workers are no longer available for a single category of clients. Still, based on the organisation's perspective of individualised help, which implies a client-focused approach (zorg op maat), the agency continues to offer group sessions for immigrant women. Moreover, the organisation recently entered into a contract-based agreement with the Central Reception Organisation for Asylum Seekers (COA) to offer psychosocial help to asylum seekers. Along with these social services, the agency also offers group sessions for refugee women in co-operation with the Organisation for the Medical Care of Asylum Seekers (MOA).

Cultural diversity in this specific social services organisation is no longer an explicit issue either in the organisation's policy reports or in its daily practice. However, some specific actions in this area have been taken. An internal study on working with immigrant clients was conducted, a migrant social worker wrote a proposal for an integral approach involving migrant women and the team participated in the training sessions on trans-cultural counselling, and the social workers working with asylum seekers and refugees were offered special education.

Anchors in Social Work Discourse

The beginnings of social services in Dutch society go back more than a hundred years. Although care for the poor already existed in the 18th century, the foundation for the first school for social work in Amsterdam in 1899 is generally considered as the symbolic milestone of the profession in the Netherlands (Waaldijk et al. 1999). Following certain definitions of professionalism (Wilensky 1964; Freidson 1986), some even assert that professional social services in the Netherlands did not actually start until after the Second World War, when social work icon Marie Kamphuis introduced the American methodological innovations of social casework. Social casework is a method and a process in which the contact and relationship between client and professional are central issues, with the aim of mobilising clients to 'better adapt' to their social contexts (Waaldijk 1999: 121).

Social work traditionally focuses on the management of everyday life (Gastelaars 1985), which in earlier times quite normatively concentrated on 'adapting the unadjusted' to the standards of 'good citizens'. Nowadays, the 'programmed change' (Van der Haar & Gastelaars 2004) proposed by social work predominantly consists of emancipation and individualisation. As social services agencies are subject to public finance and are therefore part of the wide range of street-level bureaucracies that are related to the Dutch social state (Lipsky 1980; on social workers as street level bureaucrats) government social policy also frames their practices. The current government administration defines three aims: increasing the self-realisation of people, stimulating their self-reliance, and stimulating their participation in society (Welzijnswet 1994, Art. 1. b1). A Dutch Social Employers' Group (Maatschappelijke Ondernemers Groep) dedicated to serving social welfare interests has incorporated these aims into its vision document, and expresses the public mission of social work as 'contributing to the self-reliance of people' (Maatschappelijke Ondernemers Groep 2002).[6]

The analysis of the interviews identified five anchors, referring to the practical frames of reference of social workers. The first four anchors accentuate the relational aspect of everyday social work practice. The fifth refers to the current dominant aim of social work.

The first anchor is known as the client-centred approach, in which social workers focus on the actual relationships with their clients. The ever-recurrent phrase 'linking up with where the client stands' in the social work department seems to capture this primary approach to social work practice. This is manifested in how social workers take 'the question as formulated by the client' as the starting point for their path of assistance.

The second anchor is the placing of the individual in his or her social context. Again, the organisation in this research places a lot of value on its professionals connecting with where the client stands. This anchor clearly articulates an individualising approach towards clients. One of the interviewees explained that in the contact with the client she tried to walk on his 'map' in order to 'find out how this client looks at the world'. This provided the actual starting point for her counselling efforts. In social-work jargon or formal language, terms like 'involving the client and his system', referring for example to the family, work environment or neighbourhood, are also be used to refer to this issue.

The third anchor is the mutual negotiation process between professional and client, characterised by a more or less symmetrical relation. The Dutch sociologist De Swaan (1982) defines this as a negotiation regime (onderhandelings-huishouding). In the quote below, a social worker relates explicitly to this regime, as he clearly differentiates his position from that of the traditionally highly-valued medical sector, where the image of 'people in white coats' still holds, accentuating a large distance between the professional doctor and his lay patients. He also relates this mutual negotiation process to the first two anchors, claiming to support his client.

> What we want to avoid is that we are the experts and that the client is the dependent person who asks for help... in earlier times, of course, it was the social workers, from the medical point of view they were the doctors, the men in the white coats... and as far as the one who asked for help was concerned, you were ignorant and uninformed... What we want to try is to stand next to people and look at their situations together with them, and be as non-hierarchical as possible. (Interview with social worker, 23 October 2003)

Pointing out that social workers – interestingly referred to as 'we' by this social worker – do not want their clients to be dependent on the professional serves as a direct link to the third anchor of trying to create a more or less symmetrical power relationship between the two parties. As a result of this attitude towards clients, communication between professionals and clients in the Dutch social sector tends to be non-authoritarian.

The accent of the fourth anchor lies on change in the client's situation. To be precise, social work assumes that the client will take his or her own steps during the path of assistance. This anchor also assumes a client who is motivated and actively trying to solve the defined problem. In the following quote, a social worker explains this focus on change as she talks about the client's personal development through counselling:

> You can work together with them towards a moment of development... Well, and that is what you could call social work, to develop yourself personally, even though you have doubts, personal development means making sure

you never have those doubts again... so, that is what inspires me the most in this profession. (Interview with social worker, 2 October 2003)

The fifth anchor is often labelled empowerment. The major issues here are autonomy and personal responsibility. These issues are clearly in concordance with government social policy, as described earlier. As seen in the fourth anchor, social work interventions often focus on some sort of change in the client's situation. The fifth anchor suggests that social workers prefer their interventions to follow a certain route of development, namely that of empowerment. The focus of social work is to stimulate the emancipation of the client. The following interview fragment illustrates the empowerment anchor:

> The emancipatory vision from which social work starts is making people aware of the problem, of their situation... getting people to be aware of the fact that they have their own choices, and to support them in creating a different situation, both within the person and within the situation. (Interview with social worker, 5 November 2003)

Besides the anchors, social workers also present a significantly uniform picture of what a client ought to be doing, or at least what he should be learning during the consultations and how to act in the future. Social workers compare their clients with their own representations of an ideal client. Where once the social services sector was criticised for its paternalism and patronising approach, empowerment is now central in its attitudes toward clients. According to the interviewees, the people they deal with should have or at least develop self-reflection, self-reliance, self-support, personal responsibility, awareness of one's own capabilities, awareness of the fact that people can make their own choices in life, and a network of people around them.

These definitions belong to the script of a modern responsible and autonomous individual, which is very much the current cultural framework in the Netherlands. This script dominates the agenda setting of social workers. It is within these 'codes of the ideal client' that social workers frame their contacts with individual clients. Social workers approach their immigrant clients in conformity with this characteristic repertoire.

Constructing 'Culture' as Difficult

In various ways, the everyday practice of social workers is full of dealings with diversity. The primary approach of social work, to 'place every individual in his social context', already points out the importance of differentiating between clients. Moreover, categorising and labelling clients is a routine part of the professional repertoire – although most social workers are well aware that this labelling is risky, if only because it easily leads to stigmatisation.

Despite this individualising approach, social workers quite often end up reducing 'people of another culture' – in most cases the interviewees referred to are immigrants or refugees/asylum-seekers – to a relatively homogeneous group. The general tendency of the interview responses was for social workers to experience difficulties when dealing with cultural diversity in their practice. To paraphrase from the interview material, words like difficult, tough, complex and hard (plus more positive connotations such as fascinating, nice but ambivalent and special) were used when referring to the actual social work practice. Despite these evaluations, none of the social workers would ever exclude immigrants from their caseloads.

'Specific conditions' of their migrant clients result in a dynamic of practising social work in which a considerable number of interviewees identify some sort of problem. Social workers typified their problems related to working with migrants in terms of their professional identifications, using their professional jargon or formal language. To quote again from the interviews, social workers used terms like 'somatisation of problems', 'having difficulties talking about emotional problems', 'being passive', 'having little self-reflection', 'having a victim mentality', 'being theatrical', 'being isolated', 'being limited or non-emancipated', and 'having other norms and values' (for example with regard to gender relations). Some interviewees mentioned that immigrants have 'other expectations' of social services. The following quote from an interview with a social worker who preferred not to work with immigrants illustrates these accounts:

> What I found difficult about it [dealing with migrant clients] was... the victim... mentality, making things so theatrical... I found it difficult to work with foreigners because they keep sticking in 'Oh, oh I am so pitiful' instead of what can you do about it yourself... that might seem somewhat black-and-white. (Interview with social worker, 10 November 2003)

From the interviews it appears that culture was frequently used as an explanatory category (Bulcaen & Blommaert 1999). A more relativist stance on culture was also heard in the accounts, and here I paraphrase from the interviews: 'Culture is only a packaging, or something like that... human beings do not differ fundamentally, I think... it is often about the same things' (8 October 2003); 'I think it is nonsense to say that... culture justifies everything' (22 October 2003); 'An exaggerated amount of respect for culture... you constrain people by only walking on this map' (17 October 2003). Still, on this issue, social workers generally mentioned that it was culture that made dealing with immigrants so difficult.

WHEN DIVERSITY MATTERS

Cultural differences were experienced as obstacles to their preferential social work practice. Interviewees noted that 'it is difficult to take steps', that they have to 'repeat things a lot', that you have to 'create a lot of conditions', and that they have to 'involve the context' (family, religion). The same social worker from the introductory quote explains more specifically why she experiences difficulties in her dealings with migrant women, in this case with a Turkish background. In her account, the social worker claims culture as the reason for being unable to perform as professionally as she would like:

> It is... uh... the limitations that they [she refers to women with a Turkish background] have in their culture... For example when you observe homesickness in a woman, she is very limited in all her activities because she is under her husband's thumb, which again is a cultural arrangement. Then it is very difficult for me to work on standing up for yourself or making choices of your own while that is what they want to learn, but it just is not possible because they do not get the space because of cultural aspects. (Interview with social worker, 7 October 2003)

When we look at the language that the social workers used in the interviews, in a considerable number of cases, expressions like 'that other culture', 'cultural arrangement', 'cultural boundaries', 'culture aspect', 'from their point of view', 'because of their culture', 'embedded in the culture' and 'it is so interwoven in that culture' are used to emphasise the accounts. A set of generalisations is used to define the migrant clientele, which appears to produce, at least in this part of the conversation, a picture of the migrant client as first and foremost determined and determinable by culture. At this point, it must also be said that some of the clients also use culture to explain their situations. Nonetheless, the interviewed social workers tend to classify migrants as a homogeneous group in which all of the ethnic groups take part in and appear to show the same patterns of behaviour. Thus, it is this culture thing that represents absolute 'otherness' (see also Anis 2005).

Even more specific are the accounts in which social workers use terms like 'impediment', 'barrier', 'obstacle', and 'limitation' to refer to clients' cultural identifications. These accounts emphasise that some social workers use 'the culture of the client' as a fundamental explanation, for instance, of why the counselling does not proceed the way the social worker desires, or to reduce the problem of the client to a cultural dimension. The remarkable aspect of this is that, in these accounts, culture tends to override other client identity markers, such as being a woman, a mother, a neighbour or an employee.

Besides categorising all of the various migrants into one client group[7] and labelling them as 'difficult' or as using 'their culture', the interview accounts also provide various professional classifications that are specifically attached to this client group. One example is the construction of the 'classic case of the migrant'. Transforming an individual story into a professional case (Bulcaen & Blommaert 1999: 141) serves the professional repertoire, and is rationalised in this way. But these cases also present the pitfalls of essentialism, insofar as this activity confuses the distinction between general classifications and individual characteristics. For instance, many immigrant clients are characterised as discussing their problems in a psychosomatic way, not being reflective (enough) on their own lives and not taking responsibility.

In the next quote, the social worker explains how she deals with perceived limitations in terms of culture in actual counselling talks. Having identified a divergent frame of reference between herself and the client (a woman with a Turkish background), this social worker points out that she encourages the client to formulate 'a solution herself within her own cultural boundaries'. The quote shows that the social worker not only refers to the individual, but to a cultural framework ('what we are used to in the Netherlands' versus 'your culture') in order to explain the situation (see also Wikan 2002). She also encourages the client to reflect on her points of reference, which again is consistent with the 'ideal client' perspective of stimulating, or at least focusing on, client self-reflection.

> Then I say, for example, 'Well we in the Netherlands are used to dealing with that like this, but how does it work in your culture, how would you yourself deal with this, so, again, call on their own... self-reflection. (Interview with social worker, 7 October 2003)

Although this attempt could be framed as a methodological tool to create a dialogue (after Anis 2005), in doing this, the differences in terms of cultural identification are once more confirmed. Then again, this intervention of the professional could also be interpreted as an act of proximity (gaining trust through empathy).

A second example of dealing with diversity in practice demonstrates the emphasis on bringing about a change in the client's situation: A social worker – who has experienced group work with migrant women mentions that this kind of social work is successful in the sense that the women experienced the group as pleasant and they all felt safe, and tended to return over and over again. She remarks however that this 'does not contribute to what you want to achieve'. She is referring to the social work anchor of change, when she talks about 'getting people to move' and 'to really take steps'.

> It is a pity that in the end, you get so little movement there... that it is like this again and again. I have done several groups and you see the same people coming over and over again. So you can say, well, we have really offered them something good, it is nice, it is safe, it works, but it does not contribute to what you really want to achieve. (Interview with social worker, 17 October 2003)

This focus on change and movement is an expression of how social work aims to make individuals more autonomous, active and responsible. A bit further into the interview she mentions a gymnastics club as a possible replacement for group work, if the women continue to return to social services 'without really achieving anything'. As soon as this social worker is under the impression that her professional ambition to change something in the situation of the migrant women does not work, her task is over and she prefers to hand the client over to one of her colleagues in the social sector. More explicitly, this social worker is not satisfied with just any change in the client's situation; she wants her female immigrant client to move within the context of empowerment and emancipation.

In both examples, the social workers relate professional attitude and competencies to perceptions of their culturally plural clientele. The interviewees do take 'culture' into account, and search for ways to incorporate it into their repertoires. However, by focusing on the existing social work discourse that prefers clients as modern responsible and autonomous individuals after all, they seem to constrain the space for diversity. Besides, at least in these cases, the interviewees do not take into account that social work discourse is its own cultural framework.

Conclusion

In European countries, social workers are often blamed for being culturalists. An excessive respect for different cultures, as Wikan (2002) has argued, betrays assistance-seeking citizens. This chapter shows that, although social workers often see migrants as 'others', they nevertheless encourage them to pursue the uniform goal that focuses on individual empowerment and emancipation. The moral anchors used by social workers in this study show that cultural relativism is not a dominant discourse in social work practice.

The social workers presented a significant, uniform picture of what the client ought to be doing, or at least should be learning, in the course of the counselling process. Clients are measured in terms of their empowerment and emancipation – which are defined as characteristics of individualism and liberalism. All clients are expected to feel at ease within non-hierarchical mutual negotiations, and expected to fit into the objective of being willing to 'take steps' during the path of assistance. Many migrants are perceived to have a passive attitude. This evidently conflicts with the social worker's own perception of the anchor of change. The accent on empowerment as the preferred route of change can also be interpreted as constraining the space necessary for diversity. Rarely do social workers recognise that empowerment is also a hegemonic cultural framework, which could be just as much a determinant as the 'culture' they perceive as being an obstacle in the counselling process.

Notes

1. I thank Marja Gastelaars for commenting on earlier versions.
2. See Blommaert and Bulcaen (2000) on the different dimensions of the concept of discourse.
3. Although it has to be noted that the organisation's statistics on this item are not fully reliable due to impure registration.
4. The Dutch Organisation for Statistical Research (CBS) defines immigrants (allochtonen, compared with autochtonen, or native Dutch) as 'those people with at least one parent born in a foreign country' (CBS 2004). The classification of origin also distinguishes between first and second generations, and between Western and non-Western migrants (see CBS 2004 for more specifics). Note that the four main migrant groups (Turkey, Morocco, Surinam, and the Dutch Antilles/Aruba) are classified as non-Western migrants.
5. All interviews, which lasted between 60 and 120 minutes, were taped and transcribed. The questions related to the following themes: personal motivation and frames of reference, professionalism, being a social worker in an organisation, interaction with clients, and the experience of working with a culturally plural clientele. I interviewed the social workers during working hours and within the physical setting of the social services agency.
6. The manager of the investigated organisation uses the vision document of this Dutch Employers Group as a guide for the social work policy of the organisation.
7. Although the social workers are not always that specific about what people they are referring to when they talk about migrants, the interviewees are mostly referring to 'migrant women with stress'. Even more explicitly, they are talking relatively often about women with a Turkish background. The latter is explainable by the fact that migrants of Turkish origin form a considerable group of inhabitants in the city where the research was conducted.

From Residents to Neighbours

The Making of Active Citizens in Antwerp, Belgium

Maarten Loopmans

> The fostering of an active civil society is a basic part of the politics of the third way. (Giddens 1998: 78)

In the 1990s, active citizenship and community involvement spread as core concepts in social policies across post-welfarist North-western Europe. Active citizenship has been promoted as an indispensable tool for the regulation of society, in policing and safety policies, provision of social services, welfare and health policies, and local economic development (Body-Gendrot 2003; Mayer 2003; Uitermark 2003; Cruikshank 1999; O'Malley & Palmer 1996; Rose 1996), but it has been particularly prominent in politics for the regeneration of – often urban – public space (Giddens 1998; Imrie 2004). These days, involvement, consultation, and participation are pervasive notions that emerge as a new specialisation of government, having moved from the sphere of theory and social critique into professional programs and knowledge. As a consequence, new relations between citizens, professionals and policy emerge. Active citizenship turns client-citizens into co-producers and co-deliverers of services, while the tasks of professionals increasingly shift from service delivery to the co-ordination and mediation of citizen involvement in policy programs. Community involvement has been described alternatively as a new successful technique or strategy to enhance the scope and effectiveness of government, or as a means to democratise policymaking and service provision. However, little attention has been paid so far to the new dilemmas, complexities, contradictions, and resistance in the relation between government and the governed that emerge when active citizens are 'made'; indeed, the readiness of citizens to become activated is all too often taken for granted (Flint 2002; Larner & Walters 2000).

In this chapter, the analysis of a concrete program to involve residents in the management of public space reveals the practices deployed by professionals to activate city residents and to mediate between individual needs and demands of citizens, setting collective goals. More specifically, I focus on the way these practices affect how 'activated citizens' think about themselves and their relation to their neighbourhood, city and fellow citizens, leading to potentially disturbing contradictions that provoke mixed feelings and resistance.

The subject of analysis is Opsinjoren, a policy program in Antwerp, Belgium. Opsinjoren is a branch of the Opzoomeren family, a community involvement program developed in Rotterdam in the early 1990s and subsequently exported as a 'best practice' to other Dutch cities and abroad (for instance, Copenhagen in Denmark and Genk and Antwerp in Belgium). Like its Rotterdam forerunner, Opsinjoren draws on the involvement of active neighbourhood residents in public space management to address new collective problems (aggregated under the common denominator 'liveability') that cannot be regulated efficiently 'from the centre'.

The chapter draws on empirical material collected through occasional conversations and participant observations (both as participant resident and while participating in on-the-spot visits to resident groups – called 'jury rounds' hereafter – together with Opsinjoren professionals), in-depth, semi-structured interviewing (of politicians, professionals and active residents, individually as well as in group) and analysis of written sources (newspaper articles, promotional leaflets, and internal documents of the Opsinjoren team).

The first section introduces the characteristics of the Opsinjoren program. First I outline the way Opsinjoren presents itself: The program's goal as set by the local government, the rationale for seeking out community involvement, and the practices deployed to get citizens involved. I then discuss how 'active citizens' think and feel about their involvement and relation with the local government, their neighbourhood and their neighbours. Finally, the conclusion can be read as a warning as the techniques deployed to activate citizens not only stimulate participation but also contestation. A double tension arises from the deployment of citizens for the government of public space: First, between the visions and expectations of active citizens themselves and the goal of the program; second, between the expectations of active and 'passive' residents. Managing and attenuating this double tension is and will remain a principal challenge for the professionals running the program.

Opsinjoren at Work

Opsinjoren started in Antwerp in 1997. Its name is a contraction of Opzoomeren, with the age-old nickname for Antwerp citizens, señores or sinjoren. It was funded by the then urban policy fund of the Flemish government, Social Impulse Fund (SIF), which had as one of its main purposes enhancing the quality of life in cities, particularly in the most deprived urban neighbourhoods. This is exactly the target of Opsinjoren, whose official purpose, as formulated on its website, is

> encouraging communities to take initiatives to increase the quality of life and the 'liveability' of streets and neighbourhoods. The project aims at creat-

ing and reinforcing social networks, involving them in neighbourhood management, using the creativity and activity available, and stimulating engagement of local residents, organisations and schools by rewarding them for extraordinary initiatives or activities. (http://Opsinjoren.antwerpen.be)

The Opsinjoren program offers two types of 'reward' or support for once-only activities, and two types of support for more permanent activities. The Premie op Actie (Bonus for Action) rewards and provides financial and logistic support for residents' own initiatives, while the Stedelijke Actiedagen (Urban Action Days) are specific actions organised more top-down and city-wide, in order to give greater publicity to the program and attract new active residents. Initiatives could focus on the development and maintenance of street-based social networks (e.g., street barbecues, Christmas drinks) or on enhancing the quality of the living environment (sweeping one's street, putting flowers on the window sill, etc.). After an internal evaluation in 2001, it was decided to put more emphasis on the latter goal. Opsinjoren was sometimes laughed off as a 'free party fund', so the organisation felt the need to produce more 'visible' results, i.e., cleaner, greener and safer streets. Hence the number of 'free parties' per street committee sponsored by Opsinjoren is now limited to three, and in public communication an emphasis is put on the co-production of quality neighbourhood space.

It was also decided that the program should insist on a more enduring engagement of citizens; attempts were made to turn once-a-year activities into buurtcontracten (neighbourhood contracts/BCs) and to look for straatvrijwilligers (street volunteers/SVs). BCs are contracts between the city and at least five neighbours, whereby these citizens promise to take care of the cleanliness-greenness and/or safety of a square, playground or street on a permanent basis and in close collaboration with the city departments concerned. A SV does the same, but on his own.

From its very start, the Antwerp population warmly welcomed Opsinjoren. In 1997, 3000 households participated in the first Lentepoets (Spring cleaning, the main Urban Action Day), a number that continued to rise to 9500 in 2005 (over 4% of the city's total number of households). The number of SVs rose from a mere 24 in 1999 to 553 in 2005 (De Antwerpenaar 2005). Among decision makers, Opsinjoren is equally popular. In 2003, when the Flemish government abolished the Social Impulse Fund and replaced it with the City Fund (Loopmans 2005), many social programs in Antwerp faced budget cuts or were discontinued, but the budget of Opsinjoren continued to rise unabated (compare Stad Antwerpen and OCMW Antwerpen 1997; 2000 with Stad Antwerpen 2003). Opsinjoren now has an annual budget of nearly EUR 1,100,000. Its goal is to support at least 750 different neighbourhood initiatives – a goal that was already surpassed in 2001 (Stad Antwerpen 2002).

The Opsinjoren Rationale: Together for a Liveable City

The popularity of Opsinjoren, both with citizens and politicians, can be explained by the fact that it seems to grapple successfully with problems of liveability, a concept introduced by the Social Impulse Fund in 1996. This Fund was an explicit reaction against the electoral rise of the extreme-right party, the Vlaams Blok (see Loopmans et al. 2003; De Decker et al. 2005). The electoral success of this party was linked by social scientists and political analysts to a range of 'minor' issues that provoked discontent among residents of deprived neighbourhoods, such as street litter, feelings of anomy, intercultural conflicts, vandalism and petty crime.

Liveability was introduced as a container concept that made it possible to talk about the same problems while naming them differently, and it has now become a central concept for urban governance in Antwerp. The ephemeral character of many of these 'minor incivilities' makes them difficult to tackle. Street litter, loitering, noise pollution, drug trafficking, streetwalking... most of these phenomena are not targeted effectively by traditional police actions. To throw a bag full of litter on the street only needs a second of invisibility. The Antwerp city council has deployed a huge number of workers to tackle the problem of littering (police, neighbourhood surveillants, square surveillants, specialised sweeping squads called White Tornadoes; the most recent attempt featured regular officials sworn in as 'litter controllers'), with fairly little result. As Allen (2003) has noted, the power to control directly from the centre simply does not reach widely enough in time and space.

Opsinjoren intends to solve this problem of reach by involving local residents. Instead of controlling from the centre, control is split up among hundreds of 'street volunteers' and local social networks. These informal 'inspectors' remain at their post even when the formal ones go home; Opsinjoren functions 24 hours a day, 7 days a week.

In addition, active local residents are very motivated and efficient. While professionals might first consider their own safety or are hindered by rules of politeness and competence, street volunteers do not keep their mouth shut for offenders, even though this could lead to aggressive reactions, and they sometimes find creative solutions that officials are not allowed to suggest.

> B and C run a compost park together with some other neighbours. The park is open to the local residents several days a week, the volunteers keep an eye on them putting their kitchen refuse in the right bin. But whenever the park is closed and nobody is there, children climb over the fence and make a mess. Both men proudly presented a creative solution to the problem: they planted spiky bushes around the fence and fertilised them with the compost. In no time, they had grown tall and now very efficiently deter children from climbing the fence. While we were talking to them and congratulating them for their invention, two neighbourhood surveillants turned up. 'You

are not allowed to grow spiky plants in public space, the police code states', they say. 'You should remove them'. 'But who will keep the kids from climbing the fence?' 'When we are here, we tell them not to do it. But we cannot do more than that. When we are gone, they do what they like'. (Observation on jury round, 3 September 2004)

Apart from directly controlling fellow residents, participants also enhance the functioning of city institutions. They make visible otherwise 'invisible' neighbourhoods and streets to 'distant' public services. As day-to-day observers, they see and hear more than the remote bureaucrat or politician who has to make policy.

> A great advantage of our contacts with the residents' groups is the signals we receive. Through these groups we perceive what the needs of the population are. This is very important. We constantly reorganise our sweeping plans. With these signals, we can reorient our sweeping plan more efficiently. 'Signals from the citizen' can also be used to support decisions: when there is a conflict between two departments, they can be a good argument. (Head of the Antwerp Sanitation Department, interview 24)

Through Opsinjoren-supported networks of residents, city authorities are more swiftly informed about new problem areas and about what and who provokes these problems. Politicians, various sections of the sanitation department and the local police eagerly make use of these 'eyes and ears' on the street.

In addition, Opsinjoren helps the local bureaucratic top control the work of fieldworkers. Opsinjoren has enabled residents to find a very approachable channel for all kinds of complaints about garbage collectors, neighbourhood surveillants or local police officers who are not doing their job properly, and some of the more established resident networks and street volunteers have even developed direct contacts with local top-level officials and politicians themselves.

> I not only attend their meetings, many of them have my e-mail, and in the most problematic areas I'm in touch with residents on a day-to-day basis. I get mails from residents all the time, informing me about the local situation. (Head of the Antwerp Sanitation Department, interview 24)

Luring Residents into Action

> Opsinjoren is good, because it's cash on the nail. We do something and they give us something. That's why Opsinjoren is a good service to work with. (Resident, interview 33)

Guaranteeing successful 'community governance' of public space does rely on the willingness of the population to collaborate. Hence, the main task for Opsinjoren professionals consists of motivating people and bringing them into line in order to make them deployable for increasing the liveability of the neighbourhood. Except for the material and logistic support for their activities, the core element is that when you become an Opsinjoor you attain a special position; you enter into a special relation with your city. Opsinjoren creates a distinction between active and passive residents. Two principles of distinction are applied: First, active residents are allowed to partially appropriate certain parts of public space; second, they are given exclusive access to networks of urban government, something that is very difficult for other residents and users of the neighbourhood to obtain.

The idea of making residents appropriate parts of public space so as to take more responsibility for it and exert social control over it was formulated by Oscar Newman (1972). This is also a leading principle in Opsinjoren. By allowing residents to plant and take care of a nearby flowerbed, Opsinjoren counts on the fact that they will also supervise it. The Opsinjoren coordinator formulates it as such:

> If the City does it, residents don't feel like it is theirs. It is only because the ground is drenched by their own sweat that people will say: 'that's mine, I have put a lot of effort into that, I have been thinking about it, we have organised ourselves around it. It's a part of my environment, I have put a lot of energy into it, and you are going to respect it, I will make sure you do'. (Opsinjoren coordinator, interview 1)

Opsinjoren brings volunteers in touch with the network of government institutions that are engaged in the neighbourhood, even when it considers problems that are not directly linked to the activities of Opsinjoren. Since the problem of liveability touches upon various policy domains, Opsinjoren comes in touch with a wide range of city services (the department of open space planning, street cleaning, community building and the police collaborate on a regular basis); when necessary, Opsinjoren brings them in touch with dissatisfied residents. Opsinjoren professionals function as middlemen for 'their' residents, guaranteeing a swift and efficient solution of a variety of problems.

> We cross M on the street, he volunteers at the garbage park. He immediately starts off complaining about litter. 'We need to hold another meeting, with the litter department, with Opsinjoren and with the police. The problems are huge. Last week, there was this Eastern European with a broken sports bag full of garbage. He threw it on the street. I told him, "don't, it's going to cost you 135 euros, I'll call the cops". After some quarrelling, I went to the police, but you know what? They didn't have time for me! And the Aldi shop on Ooievaar street, you should also have a talk with them too. They only

have one dustbin, and they do not always put it outside. It's a regular dump out there'. (Observation on jury round, 29 September 2004)

As mentioned previously, Opsinjoren groups also profit from their status as 'organised residents' to establish direct contacts with local officials, as well as with politicians and the media. Opsinjoren residents use their network to exert more power over their environment than other residents and users of the same space, from obtaining better service provision to agenda setting.

> I find it useful that politicians attend the parties in their neighbourhood. The people are glad to see you there. Especially when they clean up, they see it as a form of recognition. When I was an alderman, I visited these activities, and then people would speak to me and say, 'what about this neighbourhood park'? And then I would say, 'ok, what's your vision? I'll put aside 6000 euros to renovate the benches'. (Former alderman, interview 6)

Making Neighbours out of Residents

There is something deeper at play behind the professional techniques of luring calculating residents. The people behind Opsinjoren made it very clear that part of the challenge also consisted of changing the way citizens think about themselves, their relation to their living environment, and the city's government and administration. Policymakers identified the attitudes of citizens as a key problem for the Antwerp city government. Increasingly, citizens seemed to have an individualistic, 'instrumental-fiscal' relationship to the city – a relationship that culminated in a very negative attitude towards city hall. The only contact politicians and officials had with residents were through 'professional complainers'. Residents only contacted the city government to claim more services and facilities for themselves, claims that simply could not always be met. A failure to do so resulted in complaints on their inadequate provision. The problem of clean streets is illustrative:

> If everybody cleans in front of his or her house, the city is 'enormously' clean. But residents don't do this anymore. They have the attitude of 'the city should take care of it, what else do I pay taxes for?' But you can have 10,000 employees cleaning, and when residents keep throwing their cigarette butts on the street, or when kids on their way home from school throw their empty bags of crisps on the pavement, it's no use. (City official, interview 25)

Opsinjoren offered a way to circumvent this 'individualistic' type of resident and to reach out to those who still feel a collective responsibility towards their city.

The Antwerp government collectively reached out to its citizens and said 'do something yourself, instead of complaining'... The core idea of Opsinjoren was that some people in the street would take initiatives themselves... Doing things collectively for your environment, that's the basis, actually. And of course, cleaning one's street is a good and simple model. (Former alderman, interview 6)

Instead of responding to individual demands by solipsistic residents, Opsinjoren focuses on 'responsible residents', who also feel emotionally tied to at least their immediate living environment.

We need to connect people to the neighbourhoods again. Neighbourhood life was disappearing. Social networks had gone. The Catholic network had disappeared, the socialist network as well. And if you live in a neighbourhood but you do not have any social ties with it... It's a fiction to create ties with a city, but it's possible with the neighbourhood. (Former alderman, interview 6)

Opsinjoren both thrives on and tries to re-establish feelings of connectedness and shared responsibility amongst the city's residents, and between citizens and their city (see also Whitehead 2004). For Opsinjoren to be successful, people had to start thinking and feeling differently about their relation with the city, or at least with their immediate living environment. What is at stake is convincing people that they do not merely inhabit a house, but also a street, a neighbourhood in which this house is situated. A home is more than just the actual building. Only when residents are convinced that they also inhabit the area around it, will they take responsibility for it and get involved in its management. The Opsinjoren motto is 'making neighbours out of residents' (De Antwerpenaar 2005). This challenge has been articulated clearly in the speech current alderwoman Pauwels wrote for the five-year anniversary of Opsinjoren.

The street and the neighbourhood are 'an extension of our house... Hence this street, this neighbourhood is something very precious, but also something vulnerable. We have to take good care of it. For the past five years, Opsinjoren has proven that together, we, the city, but above all the residents themselves, can make a huge difference. (Stad Antwerpen 2002, p. 4)

Opsinjoren puts a great deal of effort into diffusing this 'new' mental make-up amongst Antwerp citizens. Street volunteers are honoured annually at City Hall as 'good citizens', and regular promotional campaigns call on citizens to 'do it yourself'. Since the early days of Opsinjoren, a local weekly (De Streekkrant) offers a 'cake of the month' to a 'meritorious citizen' in consultation with the Opsinjoren team. Other local and national newspapers also regularly profile Opsinjoren participants in the most glowing terms.

Neighbours vs. Residents

At first glance, it appears that Opsinjoren participants have indeed taken on the subjectivity of the 'neighbourhood resident', and now think of themselves as inhabiting a neighbourhood, not just a house somewhere in the city. This seems to be the central precondition for taking responsibility for one's living environment. When asked why people participated in Opsinjoren to take care of their neighbourhood, they invariably answered –with a sense of despair in their voice – 'because we live here!'

Many respondents claimed with pride that this was indeed a new mentality, to feel part of and responsible for a neighbourhood or a street. Opsinjoren seems to have been an important trigger.

> And then this old lady next door came up to me and said: I have lived in this house for 30 years, and it's the first time I even thought of putting a flower outside on my window sill. Nobody did it, until you moved here and started with Opsinjoren. I said: Are you serious? (Resident, interview 41)

> This is a residential street. People did not bother each other. The first year I organised a street barbecue, many of the older residents met each other for the first time. They didn't even know each other's name, while they had lived here for decades! (Resident, interview 33b)

These positive accounts on the new 'neighbour mindset' can however be countered with more contradictory statements. Especially when engagement exceeded the organisation of a street party, respondents were sometimes very clear on the fact that they actually still did not consider it their task to keep the streets clean. They were quite nostalgic about the time that city sweepers took care of it. They just 'grabbed the brush' themselves because they felt deserted by city services.

> We are moonlighters, moonlighters for the city. We do their job for nothing. If I did these kinds of things for a friend, I could be prosecuted.[1] But I am doing it for the city, and they can get away with it. (Resident, interview 42)

Also, these 'new neighbours' were seldom satisfied with the results of their own – and the city's – engagement. As people are infused with the new mentality of being a neighbour, greater personal needs seem to suddenly appear concerning their environments. Identifying with the neighbourhood and the street they live in exposes them to feelings of despair. Litter and dirt become more visible and less bearable, and the uncivil behaviour or mere inactivity of others becomes an aggression upon their private self.

> The Opsinjoren coach calls E (a 35-year-old lady) a 'tough cop' (not just be-cause she works as a police officer, I have the impression). She has a very negative attitude towards her neighbours. According to her, they do not co-operate enough. 'It's impossible to motivate the people here'. She seems very demanding to me. She complains about a neighbour's lush lavender because it is too big; they should have trimmed it. The Opsinjoren coach tries to conciliate by claiming that the sidewalk is broad enough for that. (Observation on jury round, 3 September 2004)

'Active neighbours' are disappointed about those fellow citizens who do not put a similar effort into the upkeep of their residential environment. They vent a lot of frustration about the limited engagement of others:

> In this street, residents received a basket with flowers to hang beside the door from the city. The contract stipulated that the residents water their flowers. The older lady who guides us around complains: 'I took mine away because they had torn it down'. (The Opsinjoren coach already knew about it: people had destroyed the lady's wall plaster as well. It cost some money to repair the wall and therefore she did not want to run the risk again.) 'Some people take care of it, but not all of them. When I say to them, you have to water the flowers, they say 'it rains, that's enough'. W (from the Department of Open Space Planning) says terracotta balls are useful, they absorb the water and then you only have to water the flowers every four days. 'Ok, but they do nothing. The first one over there, and those two there, they do noth-ing. I told them several times and they say yes but they do nothing. (Obser-vation on jury round, 29 September 2004)

> H (55, male) is waiting for us outside. The flowerbeds around the trees in front of his door and his neighbour's look very nice, further on it looks a little less agreeable. H tells us that he cleaned the whole street this morning, and already now (13:30), there is some litter. 'Sometimes I think, the more you clean, the more they throw on the street'. He tries, but does not succeed in keeping the whole street clean. When we ask, how many people are work-ing on it, he answers, with a grin, 'What do you think?' There are only three, while many more people had signed up to help in the beginning. The Op-sinjoren coach says it is a formidable result, with only a few people. Some of the flowerbeds are empty. She asks whether people still put their bin bags on the flowers. H claims it has not improved a bit. Further down the street we meet P, a lady in her sixties. The Opsinjoren coach congratulates her: 'The street looks very nice, thanks to the residents!' P corrects her: 'That is to say, thanks to a few of the residents '. (Observation on jury round, 3 September 2004)

Besides non-participation, active neighbours are also simply confronted by fellow residents. Their partial incorporation into government networks and the right they obtain to exert a certain level of control over 'their' public space seems to be a thorn in the side to the less 'active' residents. In the stories I recorded, reactions from others vary from disbelief to utter aggression. Some people cannot imagine that someone would do this job voluntarily and are of the opinion that the SVs are paid by the city, while others attack them verbally and sometimes physically (2). A resident of a large social housing estate in the periphery puts it bluntly:

> You cannot imagine what they shout at us. 'Stupid ass, you take away other people's jobs, etc.' (Resident, interview 42)

Pestering is a common complaint, especially amongst those who are very engaged.

> E complains that someone is obviously pestering her. 'They have already broken the mirror of my car three times. She says, 'if you stick your neck out in this neighbourhood, you get all the shit thrown at you. As a SV, you're a sitting duck'. (Observation on jury round, 29 September 2004)

The partial appropriation of public space and the apparently arbitrary control active residents exert over 'their place' in particular, provokes reactions from other residents and users.

> M (70, female) guides us around 'her' flowerbed. On her own, she cleans the statue in the middle daily and keeps an eye on it. The problems are clearly overwhelming her. The monument has been thoroughly vandalised; litter lies scattered around the dustbins... 'Dogs are a problem, people let them crap here, and when I say something, they show me a finger'. M also complains that she is pestered because she takes care of the park. 'They put oil on my window sill and pilchards on my doorstep'. We say that is not nice of them and urge her to keep it up. She will, she says. (Observation on jury round, 29 September 2004)

> Mr. B (65) complains that his neighbours across the street disagree with his gardening activities. 'They asked me when I was going to remove "these weeds"' (B is growing beds of wild flowers under the trees in his street). After a while, they turned to action: they poisoned his plants – even the tree in front of their house had died – so that they had a reason to tear them out... Mr. B sounds very sad. We all pity him. (Observation on jury round, 29 September 2004)

Confrontations by non-participating neighbours provoke conflicting feelings and thoughts in the minds of participants. This demoralises them and becomes a reason for others not to get involved in 'clean and green' streets, the core business of Opsinjoren. Many prefer to stick to low-profile street parties, often with a very small group, in order to avoid confrontations or because they do not agree with the tasks that are imposed on them. This is strikingly at odds with the goals of the Opsinjoren team, as one local Opsinjoren coach relates with some contempt:

> Here you only have parties, hardly any workers. Once at one of these parties, I suggested someone partake in the annual spring-cleaning, but she looked down at me and said: we do not want to have anything to do with that! Another group even asked me whether Opsinjoren could arrange for the city's sweeping squads to pass through their street after the party. There was always a lot of litter afterwards, they said'. (Opsinjoren coach, informal conversation)

Refraining from becoming too involved is a strategy chosen by some active neighbours to avoid burnout. As one respondent put it, as an active neighbour you must try to find a balance between 'engagement' and becoming a 'village idiot':

> I only clean once a week. I've been thinking a lot about it, but I didn't want to go around cleaning up everybody's rubbish. I just wanted a reasonably clean street for myself. (Resident, interview 29)

Conclusion: Warning

The agility with which Opsinjoren connects the impetus to action emanating from individual needs and desires for policies to solve collective social problems is the main reason why the program is considered such a success. It expands the powers of city government into areas that were formerly unattainable, by making use of self-governing people. Residents are a crucial resource to attain clean and liveable streets. Opsinjoren activates residents by promoting and building upon a greater attachment to the neighbourhood or street of residence, and giving them a greater say and control over their living environment.

The techniques deployed to stimulate civic action also provoke confrontation. A double tension lies at the base of this paradox. First, a tension exists between private needs and collective goals: those attached to their living environment indeed 'take up the broom', but this often occurs more out of a feeling of desperation rather than sense of responsibility. Participants explicitly confront what they see as an unfair division of labour between the city and its citizens. Moreover, attachment to the living environment not only stimulates action, it often increases dissatisfaction and demands, as people's expectations about that same environment change.

Consequently, tensions also occur between 'active' and 'passive' neighbours. While the first group complains about the lack of engagement or poor engagement of the latter, some passive neighbours are also dissatisfied with the special status that active neighbours receive in the public space. They defy the partial appropriation of what they regard as totally public space (defined negatively as a 'no man's land') and the 'arbitrary' control active neighbours try to exert over it.

These tensions sometimes lead to overt confrontations that provoke demoralisation amongst the participants. Indeed, sometimes the active Opsinjoor not only faces fierce reactions from others using the public space, but often has difficulties reconciling collective goals with his own self-image and purposes as well. This is where Opsinjoren seems to come against its limitations. Finding a balance between the free involvement of citizens and purposive government action through them will likely be the dominant challenge for Opsinjoren professionals in the future.

Note

1. In Belgium, you can only provide your close family with services that are normally provided for by the market or the state (e.g. housecleaning, or in this case, streetsweeping). If you do it for friends or neighbours, this could be considered as moonlighting and hence you could be prosecuted. The comparison is not absurd: The head of Opsinjoren often signs certificates for volunteers who are unemployed or on social benefits; if they cannot prove to the social services that they do voluntary work for the city, they could loose (parts of) their benefit when caught 'in action'.

Authority, Trust, Knowledge and the Public Good in Disarray

Monique Kremer and Evelien Tonkens

Over the last thirty years, welfare states have witnessed a considerable number of debates concerning the identity and power of clients of social and care services. Criticism of the authoritarian and paternalistic practices of professionals and a call for democratisation have stimulated changes in services delivery. Western countries have witnessed a trend towards more user-based services, with increased attention towards clients' wishes and demands. The clients' position towards services delivery has strengthened. This shift in power was initiated by the assumption of new roles as citizens and consumers. These roles were carved out against the older idea of clients as patients (in health care) or underprivileged (in welfare and social work). The three roles of patients, citizens, and consumers respectively correspond to the three logics of services delivery: professionalism, bureaucracy, and marketisation (Knijn 2000; Freidson 2001).

In the process of turning patients into citizens or consumers, the positions of professionals were hardly ever taken into consideration. Professionals were simply seen as the problem, as the opponents. Ironically, professionals themselves have played a prominent role in this attack on professionalism. Social workers, for instance, were the first to argue that they themselves were too powerful and paternalistic towards clients and should step back (Duyvendak 1999). Health care professionals were the main force behind the strong wave of criticism of psychiatry and mental health professionalism (Tonkens 1999). Social professionals reinforced guiding notions like autonomy and independence that fundamentally changed the client-professional relationship.

But even while professionals played a crucial role in the process that resulted in new roles for patients, such as citizens and consumers, little attention has been paid to what the corresponding new roles of professionals should be. What is the new identity of professionals and what are their tasks when clients are turned into consumers or citizens? What defines good professionals in the eyes of clients as consumers and/or citizens? Are they expected to wait passively and refrain from using their powers unless asked to by the client? Or do powerful clients need powerful professionals? While the clients have changed, no explicit new role has been defined for the professionals.

We argue that the new roles of citizens and consumers tend to create new, conflicting demands of professionals, while leaving these professionals completely in the dark as to how to cope with these demands. In this chapter we identify and analyse the unresolved issues concerning the new identities and activities of professionals. We argue that the redefinition of clients from patients to consumers and citizens demands reflection and a redefinition of the roles of professionals and the interactions between clients and professionals. We focus on four aspects of the roles of professionals that have upset by the redefinition of clients: the status of their knowledge, their authority, their orientation towards the public good, and the trust between professionals and their clients. In their new roles of citizens and consumers, clients have claimed to possess more knowledge and skills concerning their own problems.

Yet what exactly is the status of their knowledge, and how does it relate to the knowledge of professionals? The question of the authority of the professional is also under pressure. Both citizens and consumers have claimed increased control over their own lives. The authority of professionals has never been totally dismissed, but it has never been made totally clear either. Additionally, the new roles of clients have also affected the issue of trust. Clients, now considered citizens and consumers, no longer trust professionals to know best and act in their interests – yet trust is acknowledged to be a precondition for any good relationship in the care and welfare sectors.

How can new forms of trust be developed and on what basis? This is the expression of the public good. While professionals used to be considered guardians of the public good, consumers and citizens have debated this notion. In different ways they have both concluded that the notion of the public good is not very valuable, because what is most important is self-interest. They presume that professionals too are only self-interested, but at the same time criticise professionals for it. So the question of what relationship professionals should have toward the public good versus their own self-interest remains unresolved.

In this chapter we sketch the ideal types of patient, consumer and citizen, and try to formulate what kind of professional would fit each ideal type. What does this role imply for the four themes mentioned – authority, trust, knowledge and the public good? What comes to the fore is that these three client roles are highly problematic when we consider these four themes. Therefore we request a fourth role, that of co-producer or participant, which is a more recent invention and fits a fourth logic, that of democratic professionalism. The role of participant or co-producer is the most promising one, as this role allows for a good balance between professionals and clients in which both perspectives and positions are acknowledged. It is built on the strengths of both, especially when it concerns trust, knowledge and the public good.

Professionalism and its Siege

In the 1950s and 1960s, people who needed care or welfare were referred to as patients (in care and cure) or the underprivileged (social work). This fitted the ideal type of professionalism: a highly exclusionary system that excludes others – especially other workers and clients – using criteria of (abstract) knowledge and skills based on expert education and training. This claim to abstract knowledge and skills was often followed by regulations of professional, regulatory schools and associations, and finally ethical codes (Abbot 1988). Although there seems to be a constant battle about what kind of occupation can be called professional, Freidson (2001) nevertheless distinguishes five characteristics: 1) a body of knowledge and skills officially recognised as based on abstract concepts and theories, and requiring the exercise of considerable discretion; 2) an occupationally controlled division of labour; 3) an occupationally controlled labour market requiring training credentials for entry and career mobility; 4) an occupationally controlled training program associated with 'higher learning', providing an opportunity for the development of new knowledge; 5) an institutionalised 'secular calling' or vocation. This vocation is rooted in an ideology serving some transcendent value (professionals work not only for the money) as well as in institutions that embody that vocation and introduce newcomers into it. Professionals, in other words, are also defined by their desire to serve the public good and given the chance, to do so via some institutionally organised practice.

Distinctive and protected knowledge and skills as well as the secular vocation to serve the public good constitute the basis of the authority and trust of professionals. This notion of professionalism can be found in the work of Parsons (1964; 1968), who used the relationship between the professional and his patient as an exemplary case of functionalism. Parsons believed that the separate and one-sided roles of professionals and clients – the uneducated patient listens to the all-knowing expert – were necessary for successful treatment. Such professional power was necessary as it was grounded in expertise, guaranteed by professional control and, Parsons argued, offset by the trust between professional and client. Authority was based on the assumption that clients had little expertise and knowledge concerning their own situations. The solid training and expertise of professionals formed the basis for the unconditional trust of clients. The professional, in turn, trusted the patient to follow his advice. This trust has been reinforced by social institutions and symbols: professionals were well-paid, had their own control mechanisms, and were often supported by welfare states and welfare insurance schemes.

As for vocation, the trust in professionals was also based on their (alleged) commitment to the public good. Freidson's fifth feature addresses this issue. Professionals were benevolent and their main aim was to cure the sick and support the underprivileged. Consequently, social workers, doctors, and other professionals assumed an important role in the allocation of care, welfare and health services. They were supposed to serve as gatekeepers of (often costly) state interventions. Because they possessed expertise and were supposed to be benevolent, they were responsible for balancing a patient's claims with the common good.

Professionalism has been fiercely criticised since the 1970s precisely because of the Parsonian 'myth' of professionals having exclusionary knowledge and who only serve the common good. Critical professionals as well as patient movements argued that professionals at best possessed a one-sided knowledge of the problem. Professionals may possess specific scientific knowledge, but without the everyday expertise of patients they would simply be incapable of making solid diagnoses. Patients claimed that their knowledge was also crucial in the care and welfare processes. Knowledge, they claimed, does not come exclusively with training and education. The criticism of professional knowledge, led to growing doubts about professionals' trust and authority as a consequence. Patients claimed that they could study their diseases themselves, and that they had much more experience with the available services than most professionals.

In the 1970s, doubts also arose about whether the unprivileged were really underprivileged and the ill really ill. It was argued that the ones who were labelled as patients were really the only sane ones because they were close to themselves, more authentic, while it was society that was sick or crazy (Tonkens 1996; 1999).

It was also argued that professionals' commitment to the public good masks their power positions and strategies, towards both other professionals and the public. Behind the mask of servitude, critics saw the alleged enjoyment of power and self-interest. Since the late 1970s, critics like Foucault and Illich – as well as Freidson in his earlier writings – pointed to the disciplinary power of professionals. The Dutch philosopher Hans Achterhuis (1979) argued that welfare professionals were not solving or reducing social problems, but were actually creating a new market, which he called The market of welfare and happiness and was also the title of his book. Professionals were more interested in keeping their jobs than in sorting out the problems of clients and more guided by self-interest than the public good. This assault received unexpected support from both workers in the field and left-wing writers (Duyvendak 1997). Professionals, it was argued, simply reinforced the passivity and helplessness of their clients.

Because of their presumed lack of real knowledge and the pursuit of their own self-interests, professionals could no longer be trusted as guardians of the public good. To be able to break professionals' power position, patients demanded a stronger voice (by way of client councils and specific rights) as well as more exit options (by choosing their own services, their own professionals). They hoped this would function as a lever and change the nature of health and social services. The two major responses to professionalism were promoting clients as consumers and as citizens. We will start with the latter.

Claiming Rights and Accountability: Bureaucracy

Clients' organisations demanded that the interests of clients be secured by legal rights as well as via the accountability of professionals. This created a new logic of performance for clients: bureaucracy. The authority of professionals was overruled by the authority of the law. Clients defined themselves as (rather passive) citizens and, as the bearers of rights in a judicial and state context. As citizens they claimed their rights to services (access) and to good treatments and protection. A stronger voice became the dominant paradigm.

Claiming power as citizens resulted in a new provisional regime in professional organisations, such as health care and welfare. Clients gained various rights such as the right to take part in decision-making, the right to complain backed-up by official complaint procedures, and the right to legal assistance from institutions and/or the state (see also Trappenburg's contribution in this volume). As a result, clients could take their grievances to court. The degree to which these rights are implemented varies by country and sector. Since this emphasis on clients' rights emerged as a way of balancing the power of professionals, no attention was ever paid to rights of the professionals or the duties of the clients. The client-professional relationship became part of a legal regime.

This bureaucratic logic of course did create new duties for professionals, who had to develop new knowledge about legal procedures and the actions that increased the risk of being taken to court. The emphasis on clients' legal rights gradually created a whole series of procedural duties for professionals that made them more accountable and would allow them prove themselves not guilty in a trial. This performance logic institutionalises distrust between clients and professionals. Not only are clients encouraged to critically observe every step a professional takes, professionals also end up distrusting their clients (will he sue me?). Professionals may, as a consequence, actually alter their behaviour to avoid lawsuits. As one senior social worker in a British study on accountability said: 'One of my clients hung himself in the garage yesterday afternoon. The first thing I was asked was "is the file up to date?" Because it's so important that the file is up to date and nobody can be held to be responsible' (in: Banks, 2004:151).

In fact, because of this growing mistrust in risky situations, professionals may opt to no longer take on high-risk clients. This came to the fore in the Savanna case in the Netherlands, where a three-year-old girl named Savanna was found dead in the trunk of a car. Her mother and boyfriend turned out to have killed her. The investigation showed that the Child Welfare Council (kinderbescherming) had seldom intervened because it had focused more on maintaining a good relationship with the mother than on protecting the child. It was the first time in Dutch history that a public prosecutor opened a criminal investigation on a legal guardian. Could she, the guardian, be charged with culpability in the homicide when carrying out duties? The organisation for child protection services warned that this strategy could cause a backlash, as guardians already felt they were faced with great difficulties in their jobs caused by the high levels of bureaucratisation. They argued: 'Who would still dare to provide child support in the Netherlands?' Top officials argued that they feared that guardians would no longer want to work in the field any longer. The professional organisation was shocked because this pressure would make the job even tougher, considering that guardians already had excessive workloads (Trouw, 12 March 2005).

Mistrust is heightened even further by the bureaucratic procedures. With clients in the role of citizens, professionals now had to focus more on following procedures than on spending most of their time providing real help. Dutch research shows that in medical care, where accountability has become more important, medical specialists spend one quarter (26%) of their time filling out bureaucratic forms and living up to procedures. This figure was only 6%, 25 years ago (Kanters et al. 2004). This is also documented in Dutch youth care, which is known to be very bureaucratic.

Bureaucracy is also a threat to the public good. Pols (2004) shows that legal procedures can also remove the moral deliberations necessary for professional intervention. In her study of nurses and care workers in psychiatric wards, the separation of clients was sometimes considered exclusively an administrative routine – as separation is now strictly regulated – rather than as a situation that needs moral deliberation. In this sense, laws do not add morality to practice but may actually be removing some.

At the same time, it is good to remember that clients have demanded and continue to demand bureaucracy and its core values: equal rights for patients and the legal and procedural accountability of professionals. The above examples also show that the rise of the bureaucratic logic creates new tensions and dilemmas because professionals were not actually supposed to completely give up the logic of professionalism. For example, the professional maxim to do everything in one's power to help a client was still adhered to by everyone. In other words, client movements attacked the entire logic of professionalism, but at the same time were silently counting on professionals to continue with their old professional habits to some degree.

Professionals thus have to find ways to balance their professional duty to provide the specific kind and amount of care or help that each client needs, while treating all clients equally. The special treatment of one client can create a whole series of lawsuits from other clients who may legally claim that they deserve the same treatment. Conversely, and particularly in a medical context, the professional maxim of trying to refrain from medical intervention if there is no imminent danger conflicts with the bureaucratic claim that all of the treatment option that are legally available be offered. John Clarke (1998) signalled a 'dispersed managerial consciousness' whereby the calculative framework of managerialism becomes embedded in everyone who works for a particular organisation. This 'dispersed juridical consciousness' also develops when citizens take more active steps toward legal strategies such as filing complaints or going to court. This only further exacerbates the mistrust between professionals and clients. Professionals then have to protect themselves from all kinds of legal claims that may have a negative impact on their professionalism.

This indicates that, although bureaucracy is seen as a guardian of the public good, the lack of discretionary professional space is problematic. Of course the law articulates the public good. Yet, while bureaucracy puts equal treatment first, in the care and social work sectors equal treatment does not always coincide with the best quality treatment for each individual or group. Here too we find a tacit return to professional values because people often still expect professionals to make an exception for their particular situation. If they do, professionals distance themselves from the bureaucratic logic and thereby become more vulnerable concerning complaints and lawsuits. Empirical research shows that professionals in care and welfare would like to be held accountable for their behaviour (Vulto & Moree 1996; Hutschemaekers 2001; Kremer & Verplanke 2004; Banks 2004). This distinguishes them from informal carers or other lay people. But with clients as citizens, the meaning of accountability has become unclear. So has the 'public good'; is it equal treatment for all, or is it tailor-made treatment for each individual?

Also, what is the public good when some clients are better-equipped to act like citizens than others? Professionals signal that some clients have more 'bureaucratic expertise' than others. Some speak up more, perhaps thanks to being better educated. These citizens know how to manoeuvre their way through the bureaucracy or an alderman or the mayor and have their demands heard, while others have no idea how to get what they want. Some health care clients know the legal procedures by heart, while others are still grateful when a doctor pays attention to their problems. When patients are primarily classified as citizens, professionals can no longer use their discretionary space to compensate those with little bureaucratic expertise.

Clients as Consumers: The Market

The 1980s and 1990s gave rise to the ideology of the market as a new model for reforming the public sector in many welfare states. Client movements embraced the market as a saviour, hoping it would provide them with the rights of bureaucratic logic without the inconvenience of slow procedures. The market was also going to put an end to clients' dependency on professionals: its logic promised that whenever the professional service lagged behind clients' standards, the new 'consumer' could simply move to another supplier. In other words, the market ideology would skip the vices of bureaucracy but preserve its virtues – having power over the professionals. But the market has instead brought authority, trust, knowledge, and the public good into disarray.

Market logic assumes that consumers have the last word on knowledge: they know best who is the most knowledgeable. Hence consumers – also called users or choosers (Cornwall & Gaventa 2001) – possess the authority over what help or care is needed, and professionals are supposed to deliver this service. Services are then called demand-based or user-based: the demands of the client are the point of departure. Professionals and professional organisations are now compelled to compete in the care and welfare markets.

Consumerism makes vague promises that the ultimate authority will be in the hands of clients. What does this mean for professionals? How can professionals be critical of clients' behaviour if they are being directly paid by them? In many European welfare states it is increasingly possible for care clients to hire a care-giver with public money. In Britain a system of Direct Payments has come into being, in the Netherlands people in need of care can receive a Personal Budget that allows them to hire an employee. But giving clients power as consumers also raises problems. In the Netherlands people employed by a Budget holder sometimes report that they have to act against their own professional standards, as otherwise they may be fired (De Gruyter 2004). Moreover, consumerism in general allows social professionals to intervene in the lives of clients or in collective problems only if they are explicitly asked to do so. It is the consumer who decides which care or welfare is necessary. This does not mean the end of their authority, but rather a focus on negative behaviour and interventions. Professionals are not entitled to interfere, unless clients cause damage or injury (Tonkens 2002). This necessarily creates a negative dynamic in the relationship between professionals and clients, further augmenting distrust.

In practice, however, consumerism actually seriously limits the authority and knowledge of consumers. First of all, competition is not based on expertise and skills, but merely on prices. Cheap care may win, rather than the care that best fits the client's needs. Marketisation also stimulates organisational mergers to eliminate competition. Since most forms of care are scarce there is little choice anyway, as Dutch marketised child care sector proves (Marangos & Plantenga 2005; RVZ 2003). Finally, in practice it is often not the consumer who chooses but intermediaries. This is clearly the case, for example, when we look at the Dutch icon of consumerism, the Personal Budget in care.[1] Many budget holders hire organisations to choose for them and arrange their care. This has led to the development of a whole new 'market' of intermediaries, simply because choosing and organising one's own care is quite complicated.

A big caveat of consumerism in the care and welfare sectors is the fact that no one is ultimately responsible for the development of knowledge and skills. Freidson was among the first scholars to criticise professional power in the 1970s, but has since become increasingly worried about the consequences of this critique, especially the loss of knowledge and skills development. One feature of professionalism is that professionals actively invest in knowledge and safeguard its use. But when this is left to the consumers – who have tight budgets anyway – it is doubtful whether individual clients are willing to pay for professional innovation. This is evident in the practice of the Dutch Personal Budget. A quick scan of home care workers who are employed via a Personal Budget also shows that they themselves are concerned about their professional development. They not only miss the direct contact with other professionals to discuss their vocation, but they also complain about the lack of space for developing their knowledge and education. Some would prefer to improve the quality of care but lack the prospect of being able to do so because they have no opportunity to consult other professionals or train and educate themselves (Sting 2004). They have no control over the development of professional knowledge, as Freidson has warned.

Moreover, the consumer does not trust the professional as the possessor of knowledge, nor as the authority to decide how to proceed. Professionals can at best be trusted to deliver what is demanded, as clients can easily take their services elsewhere. This is particularly so in the case of personal budgets where consumers are allowed to fire professionals without the usual employer-employee relationship which allows for discussion of an employee's performance. Consumerism thus makes trust weak rendering it fragile. The continuous threat of exit options is quite a contrast to the long-term investments in a relationship and the trust that may develop over time. Mol (2004) shows the difference between what she calls the language (and logic) of markets and that of care. In market language transactions are short and finite. After the transaction, the relationship is finished. The logic of care is based on continuity and interdependence as this is crucial for trust and thereby for the quality of care (Mol 2004).

Consumerism does not leave much room for the notion of the public good either. The market renders the public good as obsolete, and not something to foster. The market presumes that if all of the actors pursue their own self-interests, this automatically results in the best outcome for everyone. Freidson also worries about the disappearance of the notion of the public good by the successful assault on professionalism. His main concern is the corrosion of morality, in other words the decline of the institutional ethics of professionalism. 'What is at risk today, and likely to be a greater risk tomorrow, is the independence of professions to choose the direction of the development of their knowledge and the uses to which it is put', Freidson (2001:14) observes. Professionals have a duty to balance the public good against the needs and demands of clients and employers. Transcendent values add moral substance to the technical content of disciplines. Professionals are obliged to be the 'moral custodians' of their disciplines (Freidson 2001: 222).

Participants and Democratic Professionalism

A new, fourth logic is gradually emerging, both in the literature and in practice. This most recent logic tries to do justice to the demand for democratisation and gives rise to the criticism of professionalism while still retaining its core public values. The new logic can be described either from the perspective of the client or the professional. With the client as the starting point, this logic can be called co-production or participation (Cawston & Barbour 2003, Cornwall & Gaventa 2001) or collaboration (Vigoda 2002).) Starting from the perspective and tasks of the professional, this same logic may be called democratic professionalism (Dzur 2004a, 2004b) or civic professionalism (Sullivan 2004).

This logic should not be mistaken for client participation as such, which is often participation without professionalism. Many current examples that focus on listening to clients surpass professionals' voices altogether. This is discernible, for instance, among client panels that have been established in care services and in interactive policymaking. The dialogue in these situations is generally somewhere between the interests of the clients and managers. Professionals are usually not part of these dialogues, and if they are, they are basically there to listen, not to participate (Pollitt 2003).

The fourth logic is an adaptation of the logic of professionalism. It shares with professionalism the idea that public services are different from bureaucracy and the market in their commitments to the public good and their 'secular calling' to values such as health, education and justice, as well as their dedication to maintaining these values in society. Knowledge and skills are also very important in this logic. But there is also a crucial difference with the standard logic of professionalism. Knowledge and skills are not exclusively owned by professionals – they are the object of a dialogue between professionals and clients. Democracy itself should be seen as an important 'higher value' that should be promoted by professionals in this logic; it is comparable to health, education, and justice. Therefore the dialogue between professionals and clients plays a crucial role in this logic at the individual, group, and collective levels. This fourth logic thus resembles professionalism because professionals are acknowledged and defined as driven by a vocation rather than by status or money (Sullivan 2004). But they can only maintain that vocation via a democratic exchange with clients.

It shares the core values of participation with professionalism, and as with professionalism, the development, maintenance, and exchange of knowledge is very important. Professionals are defined by their possession of and willingness to preserve specialised knowledge from their field. By exchanging this knowledge with others collective knowledge is cultivated. But knowledge is not only exchanged among colleagues but also with clients. Professionals explain their views and procedures, acknowledge the specific knowledge that clients possess, and come to a compromise regarding the problems and solutions. 'Traditional boundaries between expert and lay become blurred. The perceptions of participants become indispensable to providing a greater "fit" with the unique features of their situation' (Cawston & Barbour 2003: 721).

This vague idea can be made more concrete with the help of Richard Sennett's *Respect* (2003). Sennett proposes that the client acknowledge the superiority of the professional's knowledge in terms of diagnosis and treatment, while the professional should acknowledge the superiority of the client's knowledge in terms of how it feels to live with a demented husband or to live on welfare for years. Note that the boundaries here between expert and lay do not become blurred at all. On the contrary, they remain quite clear, but there is a new balance as to who is the expert and who is lay in a particular area.

Including the experiences and wishes of clients and an emphasis on professionalism are tried out in innovative ways in geriatric patient care as described by Pols (2004). Even so-called silent patients offer their opinions via an 'act of appreciation', for instance. Nurses use professional strategies to find out what these enacted appreciations are (does the person like to drink coffee or not?), and then produce situations in which silent patients can enact their wishes. The latter is what Pols labels as co-production.

Various authors have claimed that trust can be restored via dialogue and the greater openness and accountability of professionals. 'Growing and serious risks of citizen's alienation, disaffection, scepticism, and increased cynicism towards governments' can be averted 'only [by] a high level of co-operation among all parties in society' (Vigoda 2002: 538). Here too, Sennett's notion of the organisation of respect can be helpful. His model is promising when it comes to restoring trust, because he makes it clear when and how authority is delegated to whom, thereby generating more peaceful and respectful situations in which trust may flourish.

As with professionalism, democratic professionalism also considers professionals as guardians and promoters of the public good. But again, defining the public good is no longer just a task for professionals, but is shared with clients. Yet civic professionalism dictates that professionals take the initiative in this respect to keep the debate on the public good alive. This is characteristic of their vocation because they are paid to be responsible. Community workers still see their task as such and they want to be able to point out the dominant social problems in specific neighbourhoods (Duyvendak & Uitermark 2005; Kremer & Verplanke 2004).

In previous decades, however, teachers were also much more involved in articulating both social and pedagogical goals and the broader needs of society. In the new professional logic, 'professionals take public leadership in solving perceived public problems' (Sullivan 2004: 18) and 're-engage the public over the nature and value of what they do for the society at large' (Ibid). Professionals must be 'in real dialogue with their publics and open to public accountability' (Ibid: 19), thereby 'inviting public response and involvement in the profession's effort to clarify its mission and responsibilities' (Ibid.).

Within this logic, the basis of trust is different than it is within professionalism. Again, the secular calling is a reason for trust, but this is combined with the democratic dialogue sketched above, as well as with the degree to which professionals actively create this dialogue and open themselves up to accountability procedures. It is also acknowledged, however, that trust is a precondition for this dialogue and cannot be a result. The starting point of a fruitful democratic dialogue is that the different parties involved dare to trust each other and only stop doing so temporarily and for a reason – if something happens that destroys that trust. Even then, they may actively seek to restore that trust, since democracy cannot flourish without it. Therefore, all parties try to stay away from a juridical relationship, reserving this for situations of serious and irresolvable conflict.

Authority is shared, since professionals and clients recognise each other's knowledge and come to a joint understanding of the problem and a mutual solution. Clients are 'seeking greater accountability from service providers', among other things 'through increased dialogue and consultation' (Cornwall & Gaventa 2001: 9). This approach combines the strength of professionalism with the recognition of clients as knowledgeable and responsible citizens. Yet professionals have to earn their authority, which means they have to discuss their actions, not only with their clients but also with a larger audience like the public at large.

Democratic professionalism leaves space for paternalistic professional interventions; at the same time, efforts are made to debate such interventions in public and thereby gain the support of the broader politically democratic community. Democratic professionalism not only means that professionals are accountable and take a leading role in discussing the public good; it also means professionals themselves need the active and clear support of the democratically elected political elite in coping with dilemmas that cannot be solved, since this coping cannot be decided on an individual basis alone. Democratic professionalism in child protection, for instance, can only be enforced when guardians are more accountable for what they are doing, and when they receive the necessary support from a broader political debate – among professionals, clients and citizens – to help sort out the devilish dilemmas they now have to sort out by themselves. The issue of whether some particular care or welfare intervention is necessary should never be confined to the private arena (as in consumerism), even though it cannot be completely resolved, the discussion on authority has to be supported in both the public and political domains. Social professionals are part of a political and normative project (De Boer & Duyvendak 2004). This entails that the discussions between professionals and clients should be inspired, motivated and supported by the broader political and social community.

Note

1. In 2004 nearly 70,000 Dutch people received a budget to purchase the care they needed and to hire a professional of their choice. Some 10,000 of them are members of the organisation of budget holders called 'Per Saldo'. This made anti-professional sentiments obvious and this policy was the result The right-wing liberal Secretary of State, Erica Terpstra, observed upon it's the policies introduction in 1995 that 'A personal budget makes handicapped people less dependent on professionals' (in Munk 2002, 11).

PART III

PROFESSIONALS

Heroes of Health Care?

Replacing the Medical Profession in the Policy Process in the UK

Celia Davies

Not so long ago, a dozen or so people were gathered together at an invitation dinner hosted by one of Britain's think tanks and health policy research funders. As the meal drew to a close, the host invited one of the academics present to open the discussion with some prepared remarks. A lively informal discussion ensued. Among those who had remained silent for a while was a senior doctor who had been invited to participate. His comments then became a point of reference for several others in the discussion. Not long after this event, I found myself at another dinner, placed next to a government minister. Learning that much of my research was on the nursing profession, and thinking of the policy-related meetings that he had attended where both nurses and doctors were present, he asked, 'Tell me, why don't the nurses say anything?'

As someone who has written about the classic and dominant professional identity exemplified by medicine as well as about nurses, allied health professionals and patients as the 'others' who sustain this identity, I am sometimes urged to say that things have changed. In this chapter I will document a number of key changes, accepting, however, that such changes are likely to be fitful and contradictory rather than tidy and unproblematic or evenly paced and linear. Change can only be achieved reciprocally with the involvement of others (including clients and co-workers). Discursive changes and the process of embedding change into institutional forms and policy practices are likely to be out of step with each other. These are some of the themes that thread through this chapter. My concern will be with arguments about the decline of medical power now prevalent in the sociology of professions, the manner in which arguments are advanced, and the often unacknowledged theoretical baggage that accompanies them. Perhaps it is time for a change of direction.

The Decline of Medical Autonomy in the UK

There is currently a fairly widespread consensus among sociologists and policy analysts about the declining power of the medical profession. This concerns the loss of a long-enjoyed autonomy to shape the day-to-day conduct of medical work, to influence priorities in the delivery of health care, and to shape public understanding of the nature of health and public policy in the field of health. Challenges to medicine have come from governments across Europe, North America and elsewhere, in an effort to reduce health care budgets and create more efficiency in public-sector spending. They have also come from a better-informed public, more prone to question and to complain, and from the rise of social movement groups that contest the medicalisation of a range of various conditions.

Neo-liberal ideas were advanced with great tenacity throughout the 1980s and early 1990s. This was aided in the UK by the successive re-election of the conservative governments that espoused them. Over a decade and more, a pattern of health care delivery that had survived for 40 years began to change shape. Performance systems that managed the sector from the centre were implemented early on. New-style general managers with a vocabulary of business principles and business planning were introduced. Professionals found themselves surrounded by an unfamiliar discourse, challenged to attend to issues of volume, quality and performance in ways that were entirely novel. The powers of newly-constituted NHS trusts deliberately encouraged entrepreneurial activity. The foundations of New Public Management (NPM) were being laid. Armed with performance information, the new managers were to ask searching questions about what was being done and how. It was not just a question of reducing waste and working more efficiently, but of managing assets to an overall advantage, outsourcing support services, and perhaps seeing opportunities for income generation. Here and elsewhere in the public sector – in schools, policing, social services, and local government administration – welfare professionals were considered out of step; their protest was ignored. Different professions, such as auditing and accountancy, came to the fore.

Adding markets to managerialism gave the new configuration more bite. Trusts would now compete with each other to win contracts in order to provide services to their local communities. If the health authority and, in some cases, the GP as purchasers were not satisfied with the details of price volume and quality, there was a real potential that the contract would go elsewhere. With this internal market or quasi-market system in place, the potential consequences of ignoring business-like thinking became more serious. Observing three specific cases of doctors, social workers and teachers, Foster and Wilding (2000) charted legislative changes that were meant 'to bring the professions to heel' (ibid: 146.). 'Looking back', they argue,

> ...we can now see that the 1950s and 1960s were a golden age for welfare professionalism. These were the decades in which policy makers trusted professionals to shape and run the social services without "outside" interference from elected politicians, public officials or consumers. (ibid: 143-4)

Taking a detailed look at the profession of medicine, Harrison and Ahmad (2000) agreed with this analysis. They point out that arguments for the decline of dominance and autonomy can be assembled at different levels. At a micro-level, calculating the price of services in quasi-markets necessarily made medical activities much more transparent, and doctors and managers now had a mutual interest 'in ensuring the survival and prosperity of their institutions' (ibid: 134). Changes to doctors' employment contracts also gave local employers more leverage. When Labour returned to power in 1997, the trend continued. The plans for reorganising primary care challenged the GPs' power. There was a new framework for examining the quality of treatments under the banner of 'clinical governance'. There was to be a standard-setting national agency reviewing the evidence base for medical interventions, the National Institute for Clinical Excellence (NICE), the production of National Service Frameworks (NSFs) defining the pathway through care for different patient groups, and a Commission for Health Improvement to provide a rolling programme of inspection that would cover each and every trust. Altogether, stronger performance management and high-profile national targets were to hold the system together. Any such shift away from locally generated practices towards more standardised national frameworks is 'a process which necessarily weakens local professionals vis-à-vis newly created auditors' (Power 1997:109).

At a meso-level, these authors urge us to look behind the public confrontations and more at the inroads made into what had been a close corporatist arrangement between the profession and the state, with considerable scope for the interests of the profession to be upheld. Successive challenges were made to the system of distinction awards, which gave substantial discretionary additions to salaries. Changes also started to be made to a 'parallel structure' for the profession inside the Department of Health which, for example, had previously put workforce planning very much in the hands of the profession which largely determined the shape of the medical career – something that had historically worked to the advantage of doctors and to the detriment of nurses (Davies 1995:70ff). New powers to investigate complaints against GPs and legislation potentially enabling changes in professional self-regulation were also cited.

At the highest macro-level, however, these authors saw few inroads into the dominance of the biomedical model of disease, notwithstanding the Labour emphasis on primary care and on working in partnership towards improving the health status of local populations. Harrison and Ahmad attributed the lack of strong resistance within the medical profession in particular to the climate generated by high-profile allegations of medical malpractice, specifically in what has become known as the Bristol doctors' case. Poor survival rates in paediatric cardiac surgery had gone unchallenged. Parents whose babies had died protested. The press and public interest in what was the longest-running case under investigation was intense. A debate opened up as never before about how doctors behaved and how far the medical profession could be trusted to regulate its own members. While acknowledging a number of important caveats, the authors nonetheless sum up:

> The conclusion remains that for the ordinary medical clinician autonomy has been eroded... and that this is the case for high-status specialities such as surgery as for the less prestigious ones such as general practice. Thus it has increasingly become the case that doctors must adopt a managerial perspective in order to progress within the profession, and that clinical decisions must be justified by reference to external research findings. (Harrison & Ahmad 2000:138)

An Argument Extended

Evidence can be marshalled from more recent years, which ostensibly strengthens this loss-of-power thesis. First, there have been some dramatic new moves at the workplace level, focusing on the re-organisation of clinical practices and on new roles and alternative modes of delivery of care. The NHS Modernisation Agency, formed in 2001, developed a range of organisational redesign projects derived from an examination of the patient journey, and over a four-year period was particularly active in advocating radical changes in the ways in which clinical staff worked. New ideas have been cascaded out via conferences and training events and new roles are in place shifting the traditional boundaries between doctors, nurses and allied health professionals (Davies 2003).

Legislation has underpinned this change. The 2001 Health and Social Care Act gave nurses and pharmacists the right to prescribe a limited list of drugs. Demonstration projects have been funded under a 'changing workforce' banner (DOH 2002). The NHS Plan (DOH 2000b), published during the government's re-election campaign, underlined all of this, adding some strong anti-professional rhetoric. For all its praise for staff and assurances that they would have the freedom to shape the care they provided and to tailor it to individual circumstances, their relations with patients were deemed hierarchical and paternalistic. There was a reference to 'old-fashioned demarcations' and 'unnecessary boundaries' in what, in many ways, is still 'a 1940s system in a twenty-first century world' (DOH 2000b:15; see also DOH 2000a). A chapter on nurses, midwives, therapists and other NHS staff made it clear just how much central thinking there had already been on repositioning the work of the various health professions to take over the work previously within the scope of medicine. National frameworks, giving benchmarks for children's services, availability of old-age care, mental health services, renal services, and more have developed apace; so too have clinical guidelines and protocols for practice (Appleby & Coote 2002). The National Patient Safety Agency, another national-level regulator, began work on systems for reporting and controlling levels of medical error and patient safety. At the practical level, the loss-of-power thesis seems to have been further underpinned.

A second consideration concerns what has been happening recently to the collective self-regulation of the medical profession, the institutional arrangement in the UK whereby the General Medical Council (GMC), a body largely composed of medical professionals, controls admission to and removal of doctors from the certification register that gives them the right to practice. Here the loss-of-power story is both highly visible and dramatic. Legislation in 1999 created an overarching regulator charged with the responsibility of encouraging reform and greater consistency across the different regulatory bodies in health care, and despite fierce resistance, gave the government powers to alter the structures of regulatory bodies without recourse to a full debate in Parliament (see Davies & Beach 2000). Since then, a string of allegations of medical malpractice has made headline news, prompting the government to instigate public enquiries and reports following GMC decisions. With cases doubly in the public eye, political pressure encouraged a range of further measures. Detailed public attention has been directed for the first time to the scope of the problem of poor performance and the inadequacy of informal and the peer-led disciplinary machinery in the NHS (DOH 1999). A separate Clinical Assessment Authority was put in place to advise on poor performance, and if necessary to make assessments. Those on the medical register must now at intervals prove their continuing fitness to practice. Doctors who are suspended or struck from the register will now find it increasingly harder to return to the medical profession. The structure of the GMC itself has changed, with an increased proportion of lay people. Government has also taken an interest in medical education, supporting schemes for non-traditional entrants, putting pressure on the length of medical training, and developing plans for shared learning and for 'bolt-on' modules to enable other practitioners to take on specialist clinical work. All in all, the 'gentlemen's club' character of the GMC and its 'light touch' form of regulation (Stacey 1992) are barely recognisable these days.

A third important development affecting state-profession relations in health care has been the rise of organised patient and consumer groups, and government's willingness to incorporate them into the policy process at a national level (Baggott et al. 2004). The emergence into prominence of these groups has coincided with a broader ideological commitment to combat voter apathy and to find new ways of involving citizens at all levels. This relates to a conviction that in the 21st century, public services need to become more responsive and take strategies for user involvement altogether more seriously than in the past. Public policy development and newly-established regulatory agencies have started making room for patients and the public in new ways. Thus, alongside representatives from the various professions and health service management, representatives from the Stroke Association, the Alzheimers' Society, the Carers Association and others were co-signatories of the NHS Plan in 2000 and participated in the Modernisation Action Teams that preceded it. All of the NSFs have had patient representation. Consultations on clinical guidelines at NICE not only involve patient groups but offer support to enable patients to contribute. A further device, a Citizens Council, has also been tried. There is now a 'patients' czar' in a senior position at the Department of Health. In the context of what is now a strong rhetorical commitment to a patient-centred health service, the new participants at the national policy table who sit alongside the doctors cannot be dismissed. At this level too, a case can begin to be made regarding a loss of power for the doctors.

Whatever mix of factors has prompted this – shifts in expectations galvanised by the exposure of medical malpractice, changes in the social composition of the profession, perhaps together with government haste to show a return on unprecedented levels of new investment – the evidence all seems to point in the same direction. Five years after the publication of Harrison and Ahmad's analysis, their conclusions about the decline of power of the medical profession have surely been reinforced both at the level of loss of individual clinical autonomy for the doctor and at levels beyond the workplace. And yet, it is still possible to question this account, as the following section will show. Four areas of doubt are suggested

Questioning a Loss-of-Power Orthodoxy

First, while detailed empirical evidence on loss of power by doctors may be in short supply for the period of the late 1990s (Harrison & Ahmad 2000:140), studies from the earlier stages of the move towards managerialism and markets were cautious about a loss-of-power thesis. Work in which Harrison himself was involved paints a vivid picture of early hospital trusts in England, showing moves not simply to control doctors but also to involve them more directly in the new managerial regime. Seven constraints in relation to the loss-of-power thesis are identified and discussed (Harrison & Pollitt 1994:137ff), and the study ends with the image of an 'elastic net', portraying professionals and managers as 'in the middle of a period of intense bending and stretching and re-positioning' (ibid:148). Ferlie et al. (1996) considered the potential for new patterns deriving from the introduction of a private-sector model of executives and non-executive directors on hospital boards. They too deny any simple loss-of-power thesis. They argue that the picture at that point was mixed, particularly regarding the new hybrid clinical manager roles. They did envisage a possible future where competition between professionals for contracts might place strains on professional collegiality and impair collective action – but also draw attention to changes which do not remove power so much as alter the relationship between different sections within the medical profession. They concluded that one cannot substantiate the view that there has been a unidirectional shift of power from professionals to managers in health care in the UK. The evidence is complex and sometimes contradictory, demonstrating both losses and gains in different areas and at different levels of analysis. We would argue that the most accurate interpretation is that in a changing context, the profession can be seen as altering within its boundaries, for example, between specialties and adapting in novel ways (Ferlie et al. 1996:193).

Detailed studies of medical managers bear out this complexity. The issue of whether doctor-managers are 'colonising or colonised by' the world of management has by no means been settled, and at the very least, we are witnessing a 'new and more complex power dynamics' (Thorne 2002: 1515; see also McKee et al. 1999, cf; Harrison & Ahmad 2000:138). For some, re-stratification within the profession is a more important feature (Gallagher 2003; Sheaff et al. 2004).

Second, doubt still surrounds the interpretation of the emphasis on quality. While it was clear that the idea owed much to industrial models, quality is also an 'intermediate concept' (James 1994) – that is, one that can be shaped by professionals, managers or politicians. Available evidence seems to suggest that the early quality initiatives were fragmentary, limited and confusing (Davies 2000). Doctors found it easy to distance themselves from the actions of quality directors, who frequently had a nursing background. Confronted with the need to provide a medical audit, they resisted or remoulded it in the shape of research projects under their own control (Black & Thompson 1993; Harrison & Pollitt 1994). On the face of it, the New Labour quality framework (DOH 1997; 1998) was altogether harder to cast aside, bringing as it did national guidelines on clinical effectiveness, standards for service delivery and a new regime of monitoring trust performance. But this too could cut both ways. Were clinical guidelines and protocols for practice an imposition of 'cookbook medicine' from above (Miles et al. 2000) and of a regime of rationing (Appleby & Coote 2002)? Or were they useful advice for busy practitioners that, in the words of the Chief Executive of NICE, 'far from limiting clinical freedom... actually informs it' (Dillon 2001:141)? The rise of evidence-based medicine in what has become almost a new industry for the academic arm of the profession, the strong input of doctors albeit alongside others to formulate guideline, the way the Institute built on work already being undertaken by the Medical Royal Colleges, and not least of all, the careful formula that emphasises guidelines as advice, all indicate that here too a straightforward loss-of-power argument is hard to sustain. Evidence on how guidelines are handled in the local setting by doctors adds further doubt to the issue (Parker & Lawton 2000; McDonald & Harrison 2004).

Third, what should one think of the changes involving regulating the professions? Are the government-inspired measures that have changed the character of the register and the way in which it is controlled irrefutable indicators of a loss of power? The developments have been striking, but a somewhat different view of the story emerges when medicine is compared with other health professions. Where change has been all but imposed on the other health professions, there has been a protracted, behind-the-scenes period of negotiation with the doctors (Irvine 2003). A certain amount of pre-emptive action on medicine's part was visible at an early stage (Harrison & Ahmad 2000:137). Consumer groups still argue that GMC reforms do not go far enough (Kmietovicz 2004), and one close observer of developments has recently concluded that without stronger lay input 'new forms of regulation may prove simply to be a more sophisticated version of regulation by professionals themselves' (Allsop 2004:91).

Fourth, there is the matter of the changing nature of the policy community. Have doctors been squeezed out of the close corporatist relationship they previously enjoyed? Are they incapable of influencing the current government? Are today's governments more ready to defy the opinions of medical professionals? Surprisingly, little is known about the formal and informal structures and relationships that make up the health policy community in the UK. Patient groups report that their influence has grown (Baggott et al. 2004), although systematic research on how significant the many stakeholder events are and how the dynamics of potentially unequal dialogue work in practice is not yet available. Also, not much is known about shifts in the structures of the Department of Health, and their further development and significance. There are hints that informal contacts such as those that have surrounded GMC reform may continue to be important. One factor to place firmly on the other side of the loss-of-power equation is the strategy pursued by the present government that involves recruiting charismatic figures acceptable to itself and the profession to spearhead potentially controversial changes. If the medical profession has become less effective at directly blocking change, it certainly seems that its doctors are still indispensable in shaping how change will develop and in mediating ideas to colleagues. The obvious, empirically-driven way forward on the loss-of-power thesis – amassing relevant evidence, repeatedly weighing it on both sides of the argument – leaves us with uncertainties, with answers that are 'still open', 'not sure', or perhaps 'not yet'.

Towards an Alternative

Why have people had so much difficulty with this assessment of whether or not the medical profession is in decline? It would be easy to say that we just do not have sufficient data on how things are working both on the ground and at the policy level. That may be the case, but empiricism in this field, as Frankford (1997) has vigorously argued, often has unacknowledged conceptual and theoretical baggage, restrictive both in its analytical capacity and its political visions and alternative possibilities. First, the decline thesis leads us to a terrain of power as a quantity and as zero-sum. Has it been lost by one party? Has it been gained by another? At best we defer, and at worst, lose sight of questions such as: Does this set of changes shift the manner in which policy is made and reshape how we think about health care's possibilities? Does it represent a shift in identities? Does it transform doctor-patient relationships?

Second, the decline thesis operates with a strongly subject-centred and agentic notion of power. The bounded collective entities, state and professions, or state, professions and public are centre stage. Our task becomes to chart the shifting balance of power between and perhaps also within these entities. Third, the images that it calls upon are the images of war, of battles for possession, involving cold calculation and strategic manoeuvring, attempts at capture, advance and retreat. This type of language is less commonly used today than in the past – perhaps because its militarism and masculinism makes us uneasy more quickly than hitherto. But the legacy remains, particularly in the sociology of professions in the Anglo-Saxon world. We have been so thoroughly schooled in the historical 'battles for registration' and in the project of unmasking professionalism as a quest for autonomy and control. It rests in particular on that aspect of Freidson's (1972) early and influential work on professional dominance that insisted that a profession sought control over its own work. We have since taught generations of students to think that professionalism has to be seen first and foremost as a power claim. In practice, however, and for some years now, the sociology of professions has taken a different route.

Power as Constitutive and Relational

Foucault has taught us the need to separate power from agency, to see it not as a possession but as a constant flow that is constitutive of actors and relationships. In this model, power is ubiquitous and self-sustaining. It should be seen not so much as a negative and prohibitory phenomenon but rather as something that creates interlocked identities and relationships, subjects and subjected positions, and is to be understood as relational. In this sense, power is the understanding of self and other that it makes possible, and it should be studied through discourse and texts more than through the acts of an apparently sovereign state. According to this way of thinking, the post-war settlement and the bureau-professional alliance that it entailed (Clarke & Newman 1997) was not so much a granting of autonomy by the state to the profession as the constitution of a space for legitimate state action through notions of professional expertise. The shift is a significant one. It acknowledges that state and profession are mutually constitutive, and this constitution creates state power as much as professional power. While he is not influenced by Foucauldian traditions in any overt way, Moran's comparative study of what he calls 'the health care state' in the UK, the US and Germany exemplifies this way of thinking. Health care systems, he argues, 'pose problems for statecraft' (Moran 1999:5), and the national state and health care system mutually pervade each other. He believes we should not be studying health care policies but health care politics – and the governance of medicine in all cases is at the centre of this. For him, the institutions of the state and of health care and the professions are to be seen as 'wound round each other' rather than ranged against each other. In all three countries he examined, a process of destabilisation and mutual reconstitution rather than a loss of power is a key theme. He comments on this process:

> New interests are being mobilised: stable policymaking communities are being penetrated and transformed into more open, unstable networks of actors; and hierarchies that rested heavily on the deference of citizens are being transformed as that traditional deference declines. (Moran 1999:16)

Working directly with Foucauldian theorising and with an eye on the sociology of professions to which he himself contributed earlier, Johnson draws out the implication that 'the expert is not sheltered by an environing state but shares in the autonomy (sic) of the state'. Where this is the case, he argues,

> any attempt radically to separate professional experts from official definers is misconceived... doctors themselves are intimately involved in generating official definitions of reality. (Johnson 1995:13)

The analytical strategy must shift:

> We must develop ways of talking about state and professions that conceive of the relationship not as a struggle for autonomy or control but as the interplay of integrally related structures, evolving as the combined product of occupational strategies, governmental policies and shifts in public opinion. (Johnson 1995: 16)

These injunctions fell on somewhat deaf ears at the time. What would it mean to view the earlier parts of this paper through this sort of lens? We suggest two post-war settlement moments: First, the moment when the NPM took hold, reclassifying the welfare professions as part of the problem, not as part of the solution. This represented a radical re-imagining of the state where the professions were neither the state's advisors nor its providers. A new configuration of power was assembled around the accounting professions, auditing techniques, and forms of active management that would render costs transparent on the one hand, and reduce the state budget by putting welfare out to market on the other. This configuration also began to re-valorise a new and seemingly independent agent – the sovereign consumer in the marketplace who transmutes into the citizen-consumer of public services. Subsequently, and with a new political party in power, came discourses about 'the third way' and later 'modernisation'. These had strong continuities with the immediate past but also to some extent acknowledged the continuing resistance from those with loyalties to earlier ideas of public services and the welfare state, and who had antipathy towards the 'intrusion' of business principles. They also built on the ideal of a more participatory democracy, both at the national and community levels of involvement.

All this is to suggest that professionalism is constructed in and through the state's programs. Likewise, these programs are constructed in and through the professions. This has yet to be clearly spelled. The missing element has to do not so much with what professions claim, but with what they offer.

Professionalism and its Promise

What do doctors offer? Academic writing has emphasised the power claim to a point where it eclipses what it is that professions promise or offer. I would like to propose that medicine offers a two-pronged promise – operating both at the individual level of the encounter with the patient and at the collective level where doctors participate in the policy process, both locally and particularly nationally. At best, and at the individual level, the medical profession offers a release from physical and emotional suffering and in some cases an escape from death. It replaces uncertainty and fear with hope. The unbearable is dismissed or at least made bearable, and the patient is given an opportunity to rebuild a life, mend a relationship, and feel once more at peace or in control. All of this is enough for many of us to put doubt on hold, to defer to the doctor, to be passive and compliant in adopting the 'sick role'. The joking reference to 'doctor's orders' to explain and justify a lifestyle change is one acknowledgement of this. In practice, of course, medicine may be unable to perform so heroic a feat. But the knowledge that it can, and the hope that it will do so, pervades the medical encounter, and as I will indicate below, the way in which others relate to members of the profession. Medicine, in short, offers us heroes.

The profession also has reserved a hero's seat at the policy table. The doctor embodies not only a seemingly neutral expertise, but also a commitment to the values of health and health care and to the importance of health in a policy setting. Doing the best for the individual patient in the face of an array of counter-tendencies carries over into the policy context. Members of the profession are thought of as setting aside personal interests, including financial interests and self-aggrandisement to ensure appropriate treatment for their patients. Here too they represent a wish to cut a pathway through the bureaucracy with its red tape, rules and delays; to defend the patient in the face of penny-pinching government measures; to provide a buffer against the profit-seeking drug companies; and to use clinical judgement alone to assess the worth of claims in a particular case. In these ways, a doctor has more credibility than a bureaucrat, a politician, or an industry lobbyist. The hero stands between the damsel and these dragons – traversing the dangerous terrain of politics, all the time guarding the ideals of health care.

The hero identity has, of course, immensely positive consequences. Heroes attract deference and rewards of money, status and power. They carry a strong sense of personal agency and a confident belief in themselves and their personal worth compared to others. But there are also negatives. We demand more from heroes than they can realistically deliver, and our sanctions for failure can be correspondingly great. Doctors sometimes talk about the sure knowledge of uncertainty and risk that they have to bear and of the patients' denials and unwillingness to come to terms with this. Separation from and lack of intimacy with others often follows, and the burden of individual responsibility and an internalised demand for efficacy and zero error can have a strong impact on their lives (Allsop & Mulcahy 1998; West 2004). Detachment as a coping strategy can spill over into arrogance and a failure to double check their judgements and practices with others – as illustrated dramatically in some of the recent public enquiries into the actions of particular practitioners. The 'flaw of self-sufficiency' and the dynamic that can separate a group from its social context was identified long ago (Freidson 1970:368ff), but it has been only minimally heeded in current debates.

Does a much more informed, educated and confident public now outdate and supersede all of this? Sociological theory has made much in recent years of the challenge to expertise across different areas of science and social engineering (Giddens 1990, Reed 1996). Scepticism about experts has given rise to a crisis in public services and a continuing emphasis on managing performance (Clarke 2003). There is evidence, at least, of a more discerning public in the way in which individual medical practitioners have been effectively challenged for their arrogance and poor practice, in the rising numbers of complaints, and in the growing resort to complementary and alternative forms of medicine. The strength of some patient groups in directly challenging health care practices is an indicator of a change in a similar direction. But I am not entirely convinced. What all this fails to acknowledge is the emotional charge that underpins the medical encounter – a theme recently endorsed in an important paper challenging the pre-eminence of regulatory discourse in health care policy and, instead, placing trust in the foreground (Harrison & Smith 2004). People, although more critical, still seem to trust doctors. A report on a survey of patient perceptions of doctors in the UK, the US, Canada, Germany, South Africa and Japan confirmed rising expectations on the part of patients. It also discovered, however, that doctors scored themselves rather higher than patients did on attributes such as their own compassion and understanding. The gap between doctor and patient perceptions was particularly high in the UK. But the survey also found that patients still trusted doctors – the relationship emerged, rather startlingly, as second in importance only to family relationships and above relationships with co-workers and spiritual and financial advisors (Pincock 2003). Coulter's detailed evidence on the demand for shared care and the 'autonomous patient' frequently introduces cautionary notes that echo these aforementioned points (Coulter 2002; 2003). When it comes to health, I suspect we will continue to hope for heroes – without these heroes the outlook would be too bleak.

What can be provisionally said about the durability of the hope for heroes in the context of policymaking? There are similar challenges to the persona of the neutral expert, to the altruist, and particularly to the doctor as advocate – as patient groups are increasingly directly represented in policy arenas. While ultimately there is empirical work to be done in understanding policy networks and their operation, those who would argue for the reduction of medical power need to acknowledge the kinds of contradictory tendencies that have been outlined above. I suggest they also need to consider the impact of continuing, as many doctors do, in one-to-one clinical practice. This may well serve to reinforce the hero identity of doctors now operating on a national stage. When both the wish for heroes and the unstable dynamics of heroism are factored into understanding 'decline', the resulting picture is a lot less straightforward than analysts have thus far been prepared to countenance.

Discussion

All this begins to point the sociology of professions in some new directions. The first is towards the field of emotions and the potential of psychodynamic theories for further unpacking the ambivalent consequences of the construction and demolition of heroes. The argument here is not so much about the return to such approaches in clinical and professional practice in a more regulated world (Chamberlayne & Sudbury 2001; Chamberlayne et al. 2004). It is rather about removing these analytical tools from their safe place as the expertise space of named professionals (psychiatrists, social workers, mental health nurses), and turning them instead on the professionals themselves. West (2004) provides one directly relevant example in his use of biographical methods and psychoanalytical theory to explore distress in the life histories of inner-London GPs, some of whom he describes as 'enmeshed in a discourse of the doctor as omnipotent and omniscient hero', and others who struggle against this. Psycho-dynamically influenced work in re-examining issues of 'rationality, emotion and 'race' in care work organisations also points to the power of such developments (Gunaratnam & Lewis 2001).

A second important direction points to the need for the study of professionals within the national policy process. The present policy climate in the UK, as noted at the beginning of this chapter, is one in which the government has created multiple-stakeholder discussion arenas that bring together professions, service providers, officials and representatives of organised patient groups. How do these groups mutually constitute themselves and the practice that results in health policy decisions? What transformations occur when patient representatives appear at the policy table? The doctor may be dislodged without necessarily being diminished. There is empirical work to be done here and answers may well both vary considerably with the policy context and be rather unstable as new vocabularies, identities and understandings of the possible begin to emerge.

If new thinking on the profession of medicine needs to work with an alternative model of power and to acknowledge emotion in the ways suggested, there is also a third move to be made, related to social theory and its conceptualisations of change. Here it may be more helpful to work not with familiar arguments about late modernity and its declining faith in expertise (Giddens 1991; Beck 1992), but with more recent concepts of liquid modernity (Bauman 2001, 2002). Bauman challenges the fixity of institutions, arguing that if nothing solidifies into an end state, what is left (returning to the battle imagery) is an endless series of 'reconnaissance skirmishes'. 'Things today', he suggests

> are moving sideways, aslant or across rather than forward, often backward, but as a rule, the movers are unsure of their direction and the nature of successive steps is hotly contested... (Bauman 2001:137)

In an observation particularly pertinent to the argument here, he continues:

> One change starts before another has been completed, and, most importantly, the sediments and imprints of one change are not wiped clean or erased before another change starts to scatter its own. (Ibid:137)

Conclusion

The present analysis has sought to confront some of the ambiguities that continue to surround the profession of medicine. It has explored the nature of some contemporary arguments about decline, noting their strengths but also logging their inconclusiveness. It has traced this problem to an overly simplistic and overly solid model of power, going on to argue that we need to attend to the hero identity which infuses the relation of the medical profession both with the state and with the public. All this suggests that it is now perhaps time to refresh and replenish the theory of professions, to re-infuse it with an understanding not only of claims for control, but also of the nature of the promise that it offers and our ambivalent response to it. To do this, we must address the complex relationship between state and profession – conducted under the eye of a changing public, sometimes prepared to challenge, but by no means always ready to give up on the hope that the profession of medicine offers.

In this chapter I have shown that the medical profession is not so much under siege – squeezed 'between people and policy' – as that it continues to play an altogether more ambiguous role in mediating between the two. When the heroic character of this positioning is unmasked – when, or rather if, the advantages of class, gender and ethnicity are stripped away from the medical profession – I suspect that hope and fear will continue to be present and to have a profound effect upon what happens both in the consulting room and in the corridors of political power.

Tensions in Medical Work between Patients' Interests and Administrative and Organisational Constraints

Werner Vogd

The German health care system is undergoing various changes due to what is known as the third health care reform (*Gesundheitsreform*), initiated by the Social Democratic and Green Party coalition government. Obviously, one of the aims is to reduce the general cost of health services. With the slogan 'Rationalisation without Rationing' (*Rationalisierung statt Rationierung*), a transformation process is currently taking place which influences the work of medical personnel in different ways.

This particularly affects hospital doctors, who will no longer be 'captains of the ship'. New members of hospital boards will be increasingly recruited from the administrative elites. In this process, doctors will gradually lose their influence on organisational aspects, especially with respect to human resources and strategic decisions within their hospitals. The way in which physicians conduct their daily work will also be affected. From a sociological viewpoint, there seems to be an ongoing process of de-professionalisation and dissolution of the power and autonomy of the medical profession. One might think that a new kind of professionalism is emerging, because under the new conditions, expert knowledge will remain one of the most powerful resources in medical work. But as I argue further, the configuration of this expert knowledge increasingly acquires the characteristics of highly distributed knowledge. Because of this feature I propose to use the term 'medical expert' rather than 'medical professional'.

Whether this movement affects patients negatively or positively is a question that needs to be answered empirically. The decreased power of physicians may lead to more patient autonomy. However, confronted with an anonymous organisation, it will be more difficult for patients to address their needs to an individual person, like a specific doctor.

Participant Observation in German Hospitals

The following remarks are based on ethnographic studies in German hospitals focusing on medical actions and decision-making. The investigation was accomplished in the form of a panel design, which allows us to perceive how the organisational changes have affected medical work in hospitals.

In the first part of the study field research took place from 2000 to 2002, in four different types of hospital departments (abdominal surgery, oncology, clinic for psychosomatic diseases, and a general medical ward) at several institutions. In the second part of the study, a general ward and a department of abdominal surgery were revisited during 2004.

In the period between the two field research phases, hospitals in Germany were experiencing an extensive process of organisational change. On the one hand, the introduction of the new Diagnosis Related Groups (DRG) brought about a new cost-accounting structure. The basis for calculating costs is no longer length of hospital stay, but a billing system related to diagnosis. On the other hand, connected to the ongoing privatisation of hospitals, concepts of modern management (computer-based controlling, outsourcing, and centralisation of important functions) are beginning to enter hospital life. These processes may bring about significant changes in the context of medical work, as well as in the way in which medical decisions are made. I will try to reconstruct the processes of change and their interactive dynamics in a comparative analysis with three distinct levels.

On the first level, I will focus on a pre-post comparison of the medical practices and/or the different organisational forms of medical work between the two different investigation phases. The second level will involve comparing the observations and my reconstructions of the different medical disciplines and cultures. The third level contrasts the relationship between the observed practice and the reflection of this practice by the actors. The aim of this step is to elaborate on the tensions between classic medical professional *habitus* (Bourdieu 1997) and the new organisational requirements.

The comparison of these levels is structured by various common themes that occur in all of the observed wards. Identification of these themes is guided by empirical observations. Common themes are patient management, complex and complicated cases, routine cases, organisation of ward rounds, care of dying patients, etc. Because we look less at the medical details of the treatment and more at the social organisation of these processes, we are able to abstract from an individual case. In spite of the different diseases and their particularities, we will see structural homologies, and maybe with changing administrational conditions differences in the social organisation of medical work (for further methodological details, see Vogd 2005).

Even if the empirical reality of medical routine work seems extremely complex, in many cases we can identify a common theme that shapes the dynamics of decisions in the examined wards. This is a conflict between the central values of the medical profession and economic and bureaucratic rationality. Physicians at a clinical ward would like to give maximal care to their patients, but have to act according to limited re-sources (see Vogd 2004a; 2004b). In my research, I would like to find out how the introduction of Diagnosis Related Groups and new instru-ments of economic control affect the relationship of medical profes-sionals towards their organisation and the contact with their patients. These processes may change not only the contexts of medical work, but will probably influence the way in which physicians make their decisions and manage their daily work. Maybe these processes will also affect the basic characteristics of the medical profession.

The next section reviews the characteristics of the medical profession from a traditional theoretical sociological viewpoint. This is followed by a reflection on the role of the profession in modern society under the con-ditions of functional differentiation. The previous considerations will then be clarified on the basis of empirical examples from everyday life in a general medical ward of a hospital in a large city in Germany.

Professions in the Traditional Sociological Theory

In the 1930s, Carr-Saunders and Wilson (1933) defined professions by the fact that their participants control specialised intellectual techniques, which are justified by nature or jurisprudence and have to be learned during a longer training process. The professional – and Talcott Parsons (1968) follows this definition – is therefore conscious of his social re-sponsibility with respect to his client as well as to society. It is assumed that he or she acts predominantly in the interest of welfare and the pub-lic, and does not act according to individual profit interests. From the perspective of institutional power, a profession is characterised as an in-stitutionalised organisation that regulates its interests autonomously without outside interference. The medical professional himself decides on the interpretation of his knowledge and outlines the code of his pro-fessional ethics. The profession itself trains its novices and those care occupations that are traditionally subordinated to it.

From an ideological-critical viewpoint – which is especially connected with the name Eliot Freidson (1970) – the public-interest orientation of professionals was questioned and distrusted in the 1970s. The model of hierarchical distribution of knowledge, the professional dominance of physicians, and the minor role of patients and nurses was being increas-ingly criticised. The claim for more individual patient autonomy and nurses' organisational autonomy seemed to be the appropriate demand of a democratic society of individualised citizens. With headlines like 'shared decision-making' and 'informed consent', a number of health policy discourses ensued.

In spite of the political correctness of the demand for patient emanci-pation, empirical studies as well as theoretical reflections show that there are 'good' reasons to maintain the hierarchical asymmetry between doctor and patient (or nurses) (see Charles et al. 1999; Debe et al. 1996; Guadagnoli & Ward 1998; Blanchard et al. 1988; Frank 2002; Margalith & Shapiro 1997; Saake 2004: Strull et al. 1984; Verhaak et al. 2000). This functional sociological argument does not contradict the finding that well-informed patients who understand and agree with their treatments seem to recover better than very compliant patients. The author's argument is that professional practice cannot be translated into a rational discourse between two (business) partners, i.e., doctor and patient, because when faced with serious illness, medical practitioners have to act in real time.

While scientists and social scientists are relieved from the acute pressure to act and decide, and usually have enough time to reflect on things thoroughly, physicians have to act against the risk of not acting. They have to act under ambiguous conditions. Therapies may fail and sometimes there are substantial uncertainties in the diagnosis. It is crucial to note that physicians cannot delegate responsibility, and that their authority is to be maintained under conditions of lack of knowledge and uncertainty. Practical authority results not only from scientific reasoning, but also from the asymmetric logic of the practical alliance between physician and patient (see Oevermann 2000). Thus physicians have to simultaneously act as both specialists and generalists. A physician notices the patient specifically, in terms of his disease, and in a more general sense as a whole human being in his emotional, social and existential conditions. Even if the physician is not able to help the patient with his medical knowledge and the patient is going to pass away, as a professional he has to maintain the relationship with the patient and his relatives, and offer his support.

From the outlined perspective, all the paradoxes of the modern medical system – which can be summarised in the sentence 'more medicine results in more medicine' – are not primarily caused by the misuse of power and the profit interests of physicians, but more likely by an inherent characteristic of the treatment of serious illnesses in a highly functional differentiated modern society. Seen from this sociological viewpoint, the social and economic costs of modern medicine do not originate in the uncontrolled power of physicians: in fact, in line with the scientific progress of medicine, the uncertainties within the medical decision-making process also increase. More medical knowledge requires more personal authority to interpret this knowledge.

Professions Descending from their Zenith?

In the 1970s, the medical profession appeared to be a winner of the modernisation of health care services. Its positive knowledge seemed be grow limitlessly thanks to presumably unhindered medical research. Hafferty and Light (1995) therefore speak of the 'golden age of medicine'. A decade later, the social situation had led to a different picture of the medical profession. While the economic cost of further growth in the health care system seemed to be burdening the options of the modern welfare state, diverse academic elites who claimed to be in control of health care services were now suddenly speaking in a different tone of voice. The political crisis of medicine intensified with the uncontrolled increase of its consumption as a resource. Health insurance companies and health service agencies in the Federal Republic of Germany have since 1977 been obliged to cut cost-expansion politics with the goal of a stable state budget, like in other Western countries. In terms of the aim of balancing health care expenditures, the reform was not very successful.

With the German health reform laws (which appeared in three stages in 1989, 1993 and 1997), access to economic control was gradually extended over the medical sector. External controls on the plausibility and rationality of professional services by health insurers, contracts between individual hospitals and insurance companies, and other 'regulative' practices have been made possible. 'Faced with tightening revenue streams, individual [medical] specialities have taken up arms to control particular diagnostic or therapeutic modalities... A related conflict has been drawn between generalists and specialists over who should function as a legitimate source of primary health care service' (Hafferty & Light 1995: 136).

With respect to the development of medical professionalisation, another aspect must be discussed. The ongoing functional differentiation between specialists leads to a disintegration of health services. Even if the political side, especially the former coalition government of Social Democrats and the Green Party, favours the family doctor as a gatekeeper, family doctors' contribution to the health care supply has in fact decreased continually in recent decades in terms of budget and number of practitioners.

Modern health care is no longer the job of an individual professional, it is divided labour within an institution, where the responsibilities are shared among a team of physicians and nurses. Hereby patients, especially in hospitals, rarely face an individual professional who makes a decision based on his authority and with regard to the personal relationship he has with his client. Instead, patients are usually confronted with an organisation that enacts bureaucratic routines and presents various anonymous doctors in multiple contexts. We find an increase in the tailoring of medicine. As the sociologist Rudolf Stichweh (1996: 50) points out, we can see that the evolution of modern organisations leads to a decrease in influence of the professions in favour of highly organised and bureaucratised systems of experts.

The central role of the medical professional is also challenged from another angle. With the academic institutionalisation of public health and the health care economy in the 1980s and the development of evidence-based medicine (EBM), the old clinical elites have been disputed. The medical profession itself no longer holds the top positions in the various health care organisations without a challenge. Professionals in new disciplines, such as health economists, epidemiologists and health care managers are usually not well qualified to assume clinical duties. They make their decisions far away from patients, on the basis of statistical information, and 'evaluate' medical practice without contact with the daily routines in clinical wards. This new type of academic elite prefers bureaucratic and economic ways of thinking (see Hafferty & McKinlay 1993), directing its attention to a lesser extent towards clinical problems and therefore the suffering individual, and more towards administrative affairs and resource management.

In a political and economic sense, the medical profession hereby loses its traditional power. Guidelines for medical treatment, originally formulated as self-regulating instruments for the medical profession, mutate into a means of economic and political contexts, to control the economically relevant treatment parameters (Vogd 2002). For example, German legislators now determine the form and extent of post-graduate medical training. Those doctors who do not follow this rule risk losing part of their public licence (Pfadenhauer 2004). Although the contents of this training are still controlled by medical specialists, the future will reveal whether political threats will have any real effect on the work and education of physicians.

These are all indicators of the medical professional's increasing loss of significance. Individual doctors lose their power with respect to organisational affairs, while having to face the consequences of the differentiation of their discipline into many sub-disciplines. They have to work in teams and will not always have the chance to survey the entire diagnostic and therapeutic process of those patients with whom they are involved. This kind of de-professionalisation is not limited to any single country but can be observed in all of the modern industrial nations (see Hafferty & Light 1995).

From Spoken Medicine to Written Medicine

How do the changed role of the medical profession and the current restrictive economic conditions affect everyday life in hospitals? To answer this question, let us take a look at the empirical part of this study. At an internal medicine ward, an initial superficial comparison between the two different research phases (2001 vs 2004) reveals the following differences: in the first observation, 3.75 full-time resident physicians were responsible for a ward with 36 patients. Three years later, only 2.25 resident physicians were responsible for the same ward. Apart from this reduction of medical staff, the average hospital stay had decreased from 11 to 7 days.

I discovered that there is less verbal interaction between physicians nowadays. For example, handing over information on a patient's status at shift changes now tends to be done in written form. Daily hospital routines now involve significantly fewer interactions between physicians and patients. Instead of personal interaction, medical records now seem to play a major role in organising medical decision-making. We also find an increasing fragmentation and tailoring of the treatment process. Important parts of the patient's treatment, for example the question of post-stationary care, contact with social workers, and management of patient discharge, are now handed over to nurses. Doctors are no longer responsible for the treatment process as a whole. This means that modern doctors, contrary to their own professional self-description, never seem to be responsible for the 'whole patient' any more.

While uncertainties in medical decision-making would have previously been managed by finding a consensus within the medical team, it now seems that an increasing emphasis is being laid on routines, with decisions becoming more individualised at all levels. The authority of a single individual has gained more weight in dissolving uncertainty. Let us go more into detail:

> *Dr. Martin (resident physician) to the participant observer:* Now there are two doctors for the ward and then a doctor from the diagnostic department who spends a quarter of her time at this station... Sometimes one of us works alone... then sometimes things happen that are not so good... but we are not able to take care of everything.

While three years ago resident physicians examined each of their patients attentively and in detail, a careful examination is no longer possible under today's conditions. Instead, doctors now rely on the diagnosis that the admitting physicians made:

> *Dr. Martin:* now with the overtime hours... I have just as many as before... but now they are not paid for... now I work faster ... I have less time to speak with the patient... I used to always proceed with a comprehensive internal examination... now I have to trust the examination given at the admission station.

Communication between physicians is now often conducted only in written form, on the basis of a patient's record. There is usually no time to personally hand over a patient to a colleague:

> *Dr. Martin:* I now feel strong... good mood, I am going on vacation... the last day is usually very hectic... now I have to write everything down... the other doctor has to know what will need to be done on Monday... it's not like it was in the 'good old days', when we went together on ward rounds, to visit pa-

tients three days before... back then I thought it took about a week to know a patient well... today the patient is gone within a week...

Under the 'new' organisational conditions, the treatment process appears more fragmented and tailored. There is less time to spend on physician-patient interactions. Instead of personal meetings, patient records are the medium used to figure out the patient's process. Under these conditions, the physician is no longer responsible for the 'whole' patient, but only for a part within a fragmented work process. The change from personal to written communication requires a new culture of reading and writing medical scripts, to minimise mistakes during information transfer.

Sometimes it happens that a patient is released after a cardiologic intervention without being seen or examined by a resident physician on the ward. This fragmentation sometimes causes complications:

9:45 (on the ward)
Nurse: Mrs. Schmidt, the patient who had the PCTA, had to go... she was shifted from ward 15 to ward 33 because now there is a free bed...
Dr. Kranz (resident physician): Good; once again, I have released a patient I've never seen or examined.
(to the nurse) Was an electrocardiogram done?
Nurse: Yes.
(a few minutes later the electrocardiogram assistant visits the ward)
Dr. Kranz: Has Mrs. Schmidt received an electrocardiogram?
Assistant: I don't know... Shall I do one?
Dr. Kranz: Maybe one was written up in the other ward.
Assistant: I can't remember... Shall I do one?
Dr. Kranz: She is probably already gone... then we are providing a mere skeleton of medical services (*wir machen hier nur Schmalspurmedizin*).

(10:30, in the physicians' room)
Dr. Kranz: (Prepares the documents for Mrs. Schmidt, codes the diagnoses in the computer and writes the short physician's letter. The whole procedure takes only 20 minutes).
Participant observer: Was that the female patient you did not see?
Dr. Kranz: Yes.
(A few minutes later)
Nurse: We have mixed up the letters... Mrs. Schmidt has the letter for Mrs. Smitz... I have just made a copy to give the right one to the other patient.
Dr. Kranz (to the participant observer, with a wink): You may not write down what happens here... patients being released and only briefly examined... the wrong physician letter... in earlier times, I always handed over the physician letter to the patients personally and exchanged a few words with them... today there is not enough time...

In the accelerated treatment process, competencies and responsibilities are divided into smaller fragments. Highly educated physicians in particular suffer under these new conditions, because sometimes they are only observers in a process they cannot influence:

> (In the ward: Dr. Kranz, herself a cardiologist, studies the record of a patient who has arrived after an ambulant cardiologic intervention.) Resident physician Dr. Kranz: With Mr. Nahod... our patients get a mere skeleton of medical service... usually we have to measure the cardiovascular functioning of the heart before we undertake the intervention... now this is no longer performed... I always get an uncomfortable feeling when I read that the cardiovascular functioning is unknown ...
> Participant observer: You are a cardiologist?
> Dr. Kranz: Yes, this is my problem... I am only an assistant now... and in the quality assessment 'the cardiovascular functioning is always important'... when the function is low, we can achieve a lot with different types of medication... and with the PCTA, if it is too low, it can become problematic... this is the difference between theory and practice... even though it is pointed out in the studies that patients would benefit... but whether I do it now or write something in the letter to the family doctor... it is also a question of their budget ...

The division of the treatment process and the frequent shift changes produce new demands on the organisation of medical work in the ward, where the rounds made by senior and chief physicians, means that physician sometimes meet patients not known to them :

> 8:35 (In the ward)
> Resident physician Dr. Holstein: Yesterday I was alone in the ward... and then... the ward round with the chief physician... I don't know why under these [organisational] conditions... most of the patients are unknown to me.
> Participant observer: And you saw all the patients?
> Dr. Holstein: Yes, and then it was a little bit stupid... I didn't know my colleague's patients... therefore, I could only read out loud what was written in the record... but I don't know if these facts are still up-to-date... there was a patient who had received a computer tomography the day before.
> Participant observer: Mr. Manstein?
> Dr. Holstein: Yes... I remembered the X-ray pictures only vaguely.
> Participant observer: And now? Did the chief doctor make a decision?
> Dr. Holstein: He wants to inject him... this is the problem... I know nothing about the patient... how he feels, what he expects from us... I only read from the record but I am unsure whether this is reasonable or appropriate for him ...
> Participant observer: Did you check the documents of the unknown patients in the morning?

Dr. Holstein: No, I did not have the time to do this... I had to do blood samples and arrange examinations... I only read what was documented... well, I often get the hang of the subject rather quickly.

Participant observer: And to inject him, this is the decision now?
Dr. Hollstein: He (the chief physician) says 'it's a really interesting case'... however, he cannot actually decide because he does not even know the patient.

(10:30, ward round, a few weeks later)
Chief physician: With the record... now we should also look at the charts outside the patient's room... we don't have to play more stupid than we actually are... to study the record outside the room takes just as long as inside... therefore, we have a look outside now... new conditions lead to new ways of proceeding... only the difficult cases must be familiar to every doctor ... usually there are 2 to 3 of these problematic cases on the ward...
(In the patient's room)
Chief physician (to a medical student): Where is the nurse?
(The student goes to the nurses' station. A few seconds later she comes back with a nurse.)
Nurse: Good morning... my colleague is ill... we have a nurse stepping in from ward 15 who does not know the patients...
Chief physician: Well, then tell me at least that no one will come with us.

These few details of everyday life in a hospital show that physicians in modern organisations no longer get to act as professionals in the sense of the classic sociological understanding of the word. Only periodically does a physician get to build up a personal relationship with his patient. His work depends mostly on organisational, administrational and economic obligations. The lack of personal contact touches a core value of medical professionalism. It used to be that physicians knew the whole patient. Now this knowledge has become increasingly distributed across a network of different human members in a team and the non-human agents of the organisation (e.g., the medical record; see Berg 1996). On the one hand, it has to be taken into account that in an organisation of divided labour, specialised workers may fulfil their tasks in a more qualified way, e.g., nurses may be more competent at fulfilling 'sentimental' and 'emotional work' than physicians (see Strauss et al. 1997). On the other hand, the costs of the increasing fragmentation of work should be considered, e.g., the interface problem in communications between the various agents of a treatment process.

Concluding Remarks

The cited examples indicate that German hospitals are in a transitional state. The old *habitus* of the physician in a general medical ward has been massively altered. Physicians still remember that things used to be different – that there was less bureaucracy and more time for 'spoken medicine'. Sometimes doctors miss the routines and are unsure how to adjust smoothly to the new conditions. Maybe in the future they will refer more often to formal solutions, like guidelines and standardised treatment paths for common diseases. While uncertainties in medical decision-making used to be mastered by finding a consensus within the medical team, now there is less time to discuss problematic cases with colleagues. It seems that an increasing emphasis is being placed on routines, while decisions have become more individualised at all levels. The individual authority of the medical specialist has increased for purposes of eliminating uncertainty, but it is undermined by the process of standardisation and distributed knowledge between doctors, nurses and non-human agents (Latour 1994). It seems to me that hierarchy, especially the function of the head of the medical department, may acquire a new meaning in medical organisations in the future.

The organisational changes pointed out concern work at a general medical ward in particular. We also notice more pressure in surgical stations. Surgeons feel more exploited by the organisation in their daily work routines and have less time to speak with their patients, but they essentially perform the same kind of medicine as before. The situation is especially different for resident physicians of general medical wards. Besides being exploited by their organisations, they feel that their professional identity, their own medical culture, is being threatened. They no longer see themselves in the position of being able to live up to their own professional standards. From a sociological viewpoint, they are experiencing an ongoing process of de-professionalisation, a dissolution of their medical autonomy.

Physicians at hospitals are obviously under pressure due to increasing time constraints, the importance of which lies with the economic rationale. The most expensive time is the working hour of a specialist physician, so time is one of the main factors in a medical organisation under neo-liberal conditions.

The fact that hospital stays are much shorter now than in the past is not only driven by intrinsic medical developments – such as minimally invasive surgery – it is also a consequence of the rationalisation of medical work. From this perspective, the demands of extramuralisation can be primarily seen as an economically-driven trend to reduce costs compared to the insight that care at home or at specialised institutions is statistically cheaper than care in a hospital, supervised by expensive medical experts.

The long-term effects of these processes remain an open question. We have to take into account the consequences of the education of physicians, the costs of interface problems between the new health care organisations, and the costs of administration of medical services (see Woolhandler et al. 2003). We have to think about the costs of changing the established professional medical culture, as well as reflect on the new roles of patients and their relatives and of nurses in these processes.

Empowerment of Social Services Professionals

Strategies for Professionalisation and Knowledge Development

Jeroen Gradener and Marcel Spierts

Professionals in public service do not have it easy. They suffer under the constraints of government, market and managers, and are confronted with ever-higher demands that threaten their discretionary space. Freidson (2001) sees an advancing market logic in which citizens present themselves as vocal and demanding consumers who do not want to hear about the considerations and assessments that professionals normally make on the basis of their professional standards. Administrators, civil servants and managers are also constantly making higher demands on professionals that have little to do with the work itself. Standardisation and protocols resulting from this bureaucratic logic also limit professional space.

The results of research in the degree to which the discretionary space of social professionals is threatened are less clear. Jordan (2001) predicts that in the near future professionals will no longer be able to make professional judgements. Instead, they will have to service government guidelines and policies, instructions from research departments, and orders from management. Practitioners will thus become executors instead of professionals. In the Netherlands, Tonkens (2003) also concludes that professionals find themselves in the middle of a painful fissure between highly demanding citizens and officious managers.

Further research reveals that policy developments such as accountability, free-market processes and demand-oriented work have not yet acquired an urgent meaning for the practice of many social professionals. The government does want to be in charge of things by demanding accountability and threatening to use market practices, but it does not yet know where that might eventually lead. It also seems that in some parts of the social sector (like community work) things are not so bad regarding the forceful and intrusive behaviour of managers, because they usually know from practice that a professionals' space is not a trivial concern. In fact, they often try to protect it. Social professionals aren't taken aback by citizens' outspokenness. On the contrary, fostering the empowerment of citizens is one of their main tasks (Kremer & Verplanke 2004; Spierts et al. 2003). In short, although at present – at least for part of the professional group – there is no great urgency, there are indications of a creeping curtailment of professional space. Labour market studies show that the public sector scores the worst when it comes to aspects like work pressure, work conditions, job satisfaction, absenteeism, vacancies and training facilities (Van Essen et al. 2001).

Controversial Professionalism

Social professionals frequently depend on the political and public consensus concerning the necessity of social interventions. They will receive little endorsement from public opinion, are rarely applauded in public, and their professionalism is often questioned. In turn, the mistrust of outsiders translates into a low level of professional pride and low self-esteem (Gradener 2003; Spierts et al. 2003).

There is much support for the idea that, against the growing influence of market and bureaucratic logic, the logic of professionalism is in need of reinforcement (Freidson 2001; WRR 2004). The process of the professionalisation of the social professions has stalled in recent decades, however. Social professionals could use some self-esteem to set this process in motion again. This will certainly not be a simple task. It demands that we discover the most suitable strategy for strengthening the social professions. But first we would like to outline how we will discuss the problem. We believe that the nature of knowledge development is a decisive factor in determining the current position of social professions. In the next section we will sketch the dimension of knowledge development and relate it to other dimensions, to determine the degree of professionalisation among the social professions. Subsequently, we will explore possible strategies for the development of the social professions, in order to further elaborate on the conceptual and practical consequences in the area of knowledge development. And lastly, we will show that empowerment benefits social professionals when they forge alliances with experts, policymakers and managers.

The Struggle for Knowledge

Social professionals are quite capable of agreeing on the most urgent social problems. However, their own practical expertise is insufficiently articulated in the social debate. Osmond and O'Connor (2004) claim that 'in the current environment, an incapacity to articulate what we know places us at a considerable disadvantage'. Welfare workers, for instance, often note differences in interpretation concerning the kinds of problems and the nature of necessary interventions. Knowledge of and access to specific social sector target groups are deployed mainly by *solving* politically formulated problems.

By expertise of the social professions we mean a body of knowledge and skills. The question of how knowledge and skills can be strengthened at a time when the professionalism of the social professions is under mounting pressure is central here. The effectiveness and efficacy of the interventions as well as their scientific substantiation are being increasingly discussed (WRR 2004). The institutions where social professionals work, react to this pressure by giving in to market logic and submitting themselves to a new methodological stringency. This does not do justice to the complexity and contextual orientation of the social professions. By pointing out existing professionalisation practices and strategies for knowledge development in other fields, we will show that solutions are available with which the social professions can profile themselves as an independent field.

One reason for the lack of appreciation for the knowledge and skills of social professionals lies in the limited scientific status of their professions. When the knowledge areas of the social professions are measured against other scientific disciplines, Tucker (1996: 401) says:

> Extensive exchanges in recent literature about validity... and nature and focus of professional practice... reveal social work to be fragmented, [which is] a serious obstacle to its scientific growth. The basis of this analysis is the paradigm concept of Kuhn. The degree to which a scientific discipline has reached consensus over theory, methodology, techniques and problems, forms a strong indicator for the status of such a discipline.

Tucker identifies a 'continuing, unresolved' internal debate over these topics. A strong core of scientific journals is also lacking, as are a dominant philosophical internal applicability and cohesiveness. Social professions, together with their academic environment, the socio-cultural sciences, indeed seem to be the scenario of a struggle of cultural-political views that reverberate around the development of a Kuhnian-oriented epistemology. It is a struggle, among other things, between a positivistic ('first world science') (Gareau 1986; Healy & Peile 1995); a modernistic (Ungar 2004); and a more interpretative, holistic, dialogic and knowledge gathering (Peile & McCouat 2004).

The cultural-political struggle between the knowledge domains of social work appears as of yet settled into favour a positivistic vision of science. The work field predominantly stimulates scientific research on evidence-based practice. After all, at a time in which investors want to see tangible results, there is a growing call to define a clear object, a thorough process, and a SMART-formulated result. What's more, it seems that the core task of science has become the description of 'sense and nonsense' in the field. In his attempt to measure the social professions, Tucker includes the list of prophets of objectifiable and objectified social-work practices. The dominance of managerialism in the social sector (Ming-sum & Cheung 2004) enhances this process towards the objectification of professional practices. It allows 'command knowledge' (input, output, procedures) to prevail over professional knowledge. The degree to which this sort of 'knowledge development', motivated by political pressure, really strengthens the legitimacy of interventions in the social profession is debatable.

Against these control-oriented interventions – which strive for scientific legitimation – researchers like Campbell and Jovcelovitsch (2000) plead for a more contextual approach, in which social professionals learn to make their practices more explicit in terms of content, nature, dynamics and solution. This is not the same as protocolling or converting interventions into specific 'products'. On the contrary, it is about different prioritisations and a valuation of the relation between what is 'known' and what is 'doable'. The expertise of social professionals is concealed within the social-relational as a means for empowerment, in which the technically perfect application of intervention techniques is secondary. It is a plea for 'the importance of local knowledge: participation and social representations' (Campbell & Jovcelovitsch 2000). In this rearrangement of what must be known and doable, all the normative and strategic ambitions converge so that with a conscious knowledge strategy, the social professions can claim a discretionary space where they can identify social problems in personal and professional terms, and address them.

Degree of Professionalisation

To summarise, we can state that there are indeed initiatives towards knowledge development, but there is absolutely no unit of transferable theoretical knowledge and a corresponding set of methodical concepts in the sense of a systematic body of knowledge and skills obtained through research. Reflection in the social sciences takes place only sparsely, as people are afraid to 'deliver themselves' to practice. As a consequence, there is no powerful claim of one's own expertise domain in terms of a unique knowledge and expertise that are reserved for a particular professional group.

The lack of systematic knowledge development is an indication of the degree of professionalisation of the social professions. Freidson (2001) uses four other dimensions to typify the degree of professionalisation of professions. These dimensions enable us to complete the picture of the situation of the social professions:

- *Division of labour* – Social professionals themselves are not in a position to determine what precisely has to be done. In the Dutch situation, it was mainly those particular initiatives linked to the denominational pillars during the period of 'pillarisation' that ensured that the work was done properly. Gradually over time, the government and managers increasingly began to determine what needed to be done. This has placed professionals into an increasingly dependent relationship. For example, they have little influence on determining the quality standards of their own work. The fact that the profession developed from volunteer sector has not exactly contributed to its status either.

- *Labour market* – The professional group has no control over access to the labour market. In principle, anyone can call himself or herself a socio-cultural worker, youth worker, or community worker. There are no legal provisions in this respect. Formal recognition, title protection, and registration are almost nonexistent. Moreover, protected positions are not strived for either. The plea for a 'open profession' forms a connecting thread in the history of the professionalisation of the social professions. The core notion of the open profession is that access to the social professions should be of a multiple nature. Unlike most other professions, this access is not restricted to one type of training.
- *Education and training* – Professional organisations do not give professional practitioners control over access to professional training; the curriculum; continued education, which lacks a cohesive system of training programs and corresponding certifications; and professional practitioner control over this via professional organisations.
- *Professional ideology* – Social professionals work, via subsidies and funds, on objectives that continuously demand political or even moral considerations. If the legitimacy of the goals is eliminated, the flow of subsidies can simply dry up. Hence, professional ideology and professional identity are partially dependent upon the environment. Standards and norms for good professional practices have not been established. Only social workers and community workers have a professional code, which includes provisions for a number of professional ethics issues as well as sanctions for those who failure to comply.

Professionalisation Strategy

Measured against the norm of the classic professions, the degree of professionalisation of the social professions is extremely low. What are the consequences of this low degree of professionalisation? Some opt to no longer identify these practitioners as professionals, but more as executors. Because socio-cultural workers, community workers and youth workers themselves lack an academically legitimized knowledge background and powerful professional associations, the profession cannot regulate access, and seldom operates as a group of professionals but almost exclusively as salaried employees. Thus they are per definition strongly dependent on managers (Bovens 2003).

The opposite strategy consists of setting a professionalisation process in motion through which the profession can accumulate more recognition and power. This can be done via better compliance with regulations that other highly professionalised professions such as doctors and lawyers have. As soon as the profession begins to meet these requirements, it will be more clearly distinct from other professions, which will make it increasingly clear who is qualified and what those qualifications entail.

Neither option is an attractive one. The option of *de*professionalisation does not correspond with the complex societal problems that social professionals have to deal with. Reaching the most difficult groups, acting as an in-between and the shaping co-producership of citizens requires in fact high-quality professionalism. The other option contains the danger of an excessively rigid professionalisation, with the risk professionals taking over activities from citizens and connecting less to citizens' experienced problems and everyday challenges. Besides this being at odds with the notion of an 'open profession', the wish to grow into a classic profession hides the risk of looking only inwards and not focusing enough on the traffic along the boundaries between profession and society. Questions about what outsiders, politicians, the general public and social professionals may expect and how, and perhaps most of all to what degree they can meet the expectations are not asked often enough (Koenis 1993).

Is a third way for the social professions possible, and what should it look like? Etzioni (1969) saw a different social field laid out for the 'semi-professions' such as the social work professions but also teaching and nursing. The characteristics Etzioni attributed to these semi-professions also repeatedly included 'non-characteristics-yet'. Compared to the classic professions, Etzioni considered these occupations to have less status, a shorter training period, less advanced specialised knowledge, more limited autonomy and less emphasis on the confidential character of their work. In fact, 'semi' means incomplete, flawed, and imperfect in this case. Aside from the negative connotation that the designation of semi-profession invokes, the classic professions are still the standard here, so that the objective remains the same as that of the professionalisation option.

Fully-Fledged Professions: Making a Virtue out of Need

To what degree is a third way possible for the social professions in which they can develop into full-fledged professions, not on the basis of their alleged weaknesses but precisely on the basis of their strengths and uniqueness? Social professions are often accused of being vague and diffuse. Contrary to occupations like nursing or teaching, the precise content of these professions is often unclear for outsiders. The explanation lies largely in the connection between the social professions and the quotidian, and in the fact that these professions are per definition cyclically sensitive. This has significant consequences for the actions of social professionals:

- The connection with the quotidian makes social professionals visible everywhere. Compared to nurses and teachers, for example, the organisation of their space is less clear. This applies in any event to those social professionals whose work involves outreach. Community workers, for example, can be seen in the company of a group of residents inspecting the neighbourhood or at a sports club discussing the inclusion of a group of youth. For professionals working at a specific accommodation, the use of space is different than that of a teacher or nurse.
- Practically the same applies in terms of organising time. Social professionals are less bound to fixed times. Youth workers, for example, often have to adjust their working hours to the leisure-time patterns of youth, in order to come into contact with them.
- The social order is more diffuse. Nurse-patient or teacher-pupil contacts have a social relationship between them that is fairly accurate in its delimitations and arrangement, whereas for social professionals and users of these services things tend to be far more open. There are also different degrees of involvement, varying from volunteer to the simple user of services and all sorts of co-producership forms in between.
- A fourth aspect in which the vagueness and diffuseness are manifest concerns the order and goals that are established. In education, those goals are largely set in the form of finishing levels, and the way that school life is ordered is more or less directly derived from this. Content and goals in the social professions are per definition strongly determined by professional and societal cycles. One minute a social professional may be required to combat youth disturbances, followed not much later by a request to shift his or her attention to assisting work trajectories or make parental involvement at schools a priority. The profession is thus dependent on others (politicians and managers, other financiers), who determine the social agenda.
- The fifth aspect relates to the nature of the services. Services of social professionals never involve a clear demand or supply. What is asked and what is offered are always subject to multiple interpretations. Users seldom know precisely what they want, and professionals have to make continuous efforts to understand their own intentions and discover what the problems and needs of the users are. Supply and demand are always 'mediated' in different ways. This requires normative choices that seldom or never allow the formulation of clear answers to clear questions (Kuypers 1993).

These characteristics of the work of social professionals have distinctive disadvantages, such as the image of vagueness and diffuseness it invokes in outsiders. The work also depends to a high degree on third parties and context, and requires a permanent debate about related goals. This undoubtedly has an influence on the professional identity and recognition of the social professions. There is another side to this: The social professions are usually in line with societal topicality, which obviously offers many plusses. A sensitivity to what is current, linked to the flexible way in which they deal with ordering space, time and social relationships, makes them versatile in many ways. Social professionals often function as the boosters of social innovation. Herein lies the strength and uniqueness of the social professions. They have a considerable head start when it comes to complex and unexpected situations that demand creative interventions.

Towards a Cohesive Development of Knowledge and Practice

What does a professionalisation strategy look like for the social professions taking into account the specific features that are sketched above? First, it is important to determine that the five dimensions of the logic of professionalism distinguished by Freidson are assessed differently for the social professions. The dimensions of division of labour and the labour market are less important to them. A professionalisation strategy that offers a one-sided dedication to professional group formation in order to control the division of labour and the labour market is of no use to them. It can even be a negative thing for a particular profession to pursue recognition, status and power in this way. The three remaining dimensions offer more reassurance for the development of a profession and practice. At this moment, two contributing strategies are basically manifest: evidence-based practice, and the clarification and development of practical knowledge.

Evidence-Based Practice: A Scientific Hallmark

Proponents of an evidence-based approach have pleaded that those working in the social sector should use more scientifically tested methods. In their opinion, evidence-based practice will convince not only patrons and subsidisers of the quality of the work but also entitle the clients of the social sector to be helped according to the latest insights. Evidence-based work comes from the medical sector and points to the conscious, explicit and judicious use of the best evidence available (Hutschemaekers 2001; Melief 2004). This definition still leaves room for a professional's own judgment. However, this original point of departure has been abandoned in health care practice. The meaning of evidence-based medicine nowadays is mainly the application of interventions that have been shown to be effective.

In the welfare sector, evidence-based practice has seldom been applied up to now. Some general work methods are accepted in the sense that they are described in handbooks, but they usually have not been tested externally. In practice, there is a lot of implicit use of methods, and this tends to depend on the person. Methods are generally not clearly described according to acknowledged standards (Garretsen et al. 2003).

Practical Knowledge

A second strategy to develop a profession and practice consists of recognising the value of practical knowledge, which implies an accumulated and integrated body of knowledge, views and values related to the practice a professional builds on the basis of personal and professional experience (Hutschemaekers 2001). Practical knowledge tends to be implicit and personal; contrary to what we saw in the evidence-based approach, this is not negatively valued per definition. On the contrary, the challenge of this approach consists precisely in stimulating professionals to clarify, deepen and improve their implicit and personal knowledge through exchange and dialogue. This approach implies that the renewal must thus come from the inside. Professionals must regain their trust in their own expertise. They must make their practical knowledge explicit by sharing it with each other. This is not a sinecure, given that practical knowledge is largely context-specific and hence not simple to convey. In addition, professionals are not always used to putting their knowledge into words.

Social Professions' Own Knowledge Domain

At first glance, the two aforementioned strategies seem to be opposites, but they are not irreconcilable. In fact, a cohesive development of profession and practice requires a co-ordination between the two. To this end, two-way traffic is required: both knowledge and ideas 'from the outside' and 'from the inside' should be taken advantage of and interacted upon as much as possible. However, that necessitates a different idea about knowledge and its development than is common in the evidence-based approach. Evidence-based practice places context between parentheses, and ends up being far too oriented towards application, protocol and standardisation. This is how health care professionals experience working via guidelines and standards in a top-down approach. This ultimately creates a schism between scientists and professionals. For example, guidelines and standards in family practice, where they have been used for some time now, are only followed to a limited degree (Hutschemaekers 2001).

The social professions thus require a particular approach to knowledge and development. In that sense, they can be seen as an independent knowledge domain, with a unique, recognisable body of knowledge. Even though the development of this body of knowledge is in its origin and nature related to the existing social sciences, as a field of knowledge the social professions nonetheless distinguish themselves explicitly from the scientific study of the social realm. The field of knowledge exclusively embodies the empowerment aspects of the relations between the social professional, the client(-systems) and the socio-cultural environment. What type of knowledge development is the most appropriate for that specific knowledge domain? We believe that, for now, two features are essential.

First, knowledge development within the social professions is not just some scientific strategy. The input is not the *generalisation* of knowledge and the protocolling of practical knowledge. On the contrary, it is about *specifying* social practices in their context and the social, cultural, political and economic powers that prevent people from finding their objective. One example is the issue of immigrant integration. For politicians, administrators and policymakers migrant integration is a measurable concept that is expressed mainly in speaking Dutch and the chance of participating in the labour process. Social professionals view this more contextually as a process and not so much as an end. For older immigrants it is more of an interpretation issue, compared to youth, for whom acquiring social capital (education, networking, income) is more central. In these times of hardening attitudes towards immigrant issues, this analysis gets very little attention. Knowledge of and access to the specific target groups of the social sector are deployed mainly to *solve* politically formulated problems.

Second, knowledge development relates primarily to the relationships that social professionals enter into with clients – as individuals, as a group, or as a community. It is the result of the development of a 'consensual domain' (Baerveldt 1999) in which professional and client systems work together in a dialogical manner on shared insights into the situation with regard to origin, nature and solution of the problem. This is an issue of what might be called professional artistry. The knowledge development that occurs within the consensual domain can be best described as a dance or as jamming (Healy & Peile 1995) between the social professional and the client (group). A hidden aspect is where to find the instrument of empowerment. Even if you have shared knowledge, but no lifeline to 'what the subject wants/can' you cannot make much progress as a social professional.

An Analytical Point of Departure

John Pickstone offers insight into science, technology and medicine (STM) that constitutes a possible approach toward knowledge development that fits into the social practices and interactions that take place within these practices. In his *Ways of Knowing* (2000), Pickstone described patterns of knowledge development on the basis of the history of knowledge domains such as biology, technique and medical science during the Renaissance. He does this by not only unravelling the representations of knowledge, but also by pointing out the products they create and the specific context this takes place in. For these knowledge domains, Pickstone distinguishes four strategies that read like historical phases in the cycle of knowledge development: natural history, analysis, composition of the known, and experimentation and invention. For the social professions, it is primarily the first two that are important.

Natural history describes and delimits a specific area of phenomena as perceived by a researcher. This appears to be a question of pure exploration and classification. For a social worker assisting a client with debts, at first glance a marriage crisis or a broken car engine would not fall within the knowledge domain of his intervention. In practice, the social worker would notice that a psychosocial problem – mostly also through the connection that the client himself establishes – influences the debt problem. In the end, the social worker together with the person in need will look for a connection between the relational and the financial problems, giving significance to the specific request for help. After all, the fact that car problems are not that relevant to the solution of the debt problem and therefore remains outside the description of the problem is debatable – there is something arbitrary about it. In practice, social professionals often have difficulty with the validation of such a selection of phenomena that supposedly belong or do not belong within the request for help. They tend to point to the fact that they have executed the problem exploration together with the person in need – intersubjectively, and partly constituted in a specific context, without a scientific substantiation of the chosen delimitation. According to Pickstone, however, this process of delimitation in knowledge development is universal and oriented towards 'making meanings and doing readings'. The delimitation and description of the corresponding domain leads to 'symbolic understanding' within a 'meaningful cosmos' (Pickstone 2000: 37).

Analysis and rationalisation, the second step in knowledge development, is the search for order. Pickstone (2000: 88) illustrates this strategy with an example from physicians: 'Those who mechanised the world picture separated the primary qualities of matter and motion from secondary qualities such as colour. They separated the "elements" of a successful analytical programme from those qualities which seemed less tractable, not least because they were hard to quantify'. Hereby he also points to the selective aspect of analysis, in which certain signals that are difficult to 'place' are excluded. For example, when analysing a social problem, social workers will rapidly make the sub-classification of living world and system world. Without taking into account that such an analytical distinction in fact explains very little – at best it clarifies – the parallel with the Pickstone example is easily established. Taxonomy arises of a social-societal problem when a community worker can explain the tension between a family with multiple problems and fellow neighbourhood residents in terms of intra-psychic causes (emotional deprivation), policy aspects (allocation of rental dwellings in a neighbourhood) and cultural factors (decreased tolerance for deviant behaviour). It offers clues for interventions that include for the intra-psychological dimension, talk therapy; for ineffective residential policies, influencing policy; for working on tolerance at a meso level, neighbourhood-oriented projects.

When it comes to determining more accurately the knowledge domain of the social professions, natural history and analysis are eminently important. This is an excellent normative activity. Do we opt for a delimitation of the knowledge domain in which the actions of the social professional and the problems of the client are central? To what degree does the professional use 'general interest', the concerns of politics and policy, or chooses them as points of departure in the problem description? Pickstone asserts that describing and analysing the domain of knowledge is not a rational activity but one of involvement, intentional behaviour and meaning giving.

Pickstone's observation that defining and thus also appropriating natural phenomena into a specific knowledge domain – also in the 'hard' sciences like the natural sciences and medicine – does not have a definitive theoretical foundation but one of intention and intuition, is therefore highly relevant. It shows the essentially coincidental and arbitrary character of theoretical canons, and tempts us to implement the distinction between knowledge and practice less stringently. It emancipates the problem-defining practice within social work. The normative dimension, the delimitation and identification of phenomena that belong to the socio-cultural domain, is an indispensable link of the chain of knowledge development. The 'social' is and must be wider, more diverse and more gradated because it has a different practical and normative focus than the 'academic' social disciplines, on the one hand, because its knowledge objectives have per definition a social, historical, and cultural colouring; on the other, because individuals, groups, and other connections themselves also produce the social, historical and cultural reality (Schweder 1990).

Knowledge development seen as natural history and analysis also lends itself pre-eminently to the empowerment of social professionals. In the social sector, it is mostly application-oriented knowledge practices (in Pickstone's terms, 'composition of the known', and 'experimentation and invention') that tend to predominate these days. Consequently, we see that in product development and innovation, or in making product agreements between the government and welfare agencies, the knowledge and experience of professionals play only a marginal role. Natural history and analysis are unjustly seen as marginal activities that do not contribute to market expansion and legitimation, limit application, and are difficult to test through actions.

The training of social professionals places a strong emphasis on application of methods and techniques, whereas there too description and analysis would be more adequate. It is not the problems of citizens or politicians that should lead actions, but the problem definition that the profession itself develops, in dialogue with society's interested parties. Additionally, explaining societal issues in relation to legal procedures as well as the economic and political power fields are a 'way of knowing' that make social professionals more aware of the meaning and scope of their professional actions (analysis). It is precisely the fact that the knowledge domain of social work is relational as well as socially-culturally situated and constructed, that makes this necessary if it wants to profile itself as a profession that is expert in societal discussions.

All of this brings us to another possible prioritisation of knowledge practices in the social sector. We let go of the difference between theory and practice for the sake of developing a unique epistemology in which description, analysis, practice development and renewal can be listed in terms of primary and secondary 'ways of knowing'. Is the social professional no longer served by strongly developed primary ways of knowing (delimitation, unravelling, analysis)? Knowing how to act (method, knowledge transfer) as secondary ways of knowing are suitable here. The American psychologist William James once aptly said, 'A great many people think they are thinking, while they are just rearranging their prejudices'. It is because too many people believe they understand the social domain, that we need a profession that gathers knowledge about the social world of people from the realisation that this is a superior social activity.

Prompting Knowledge Development in Practice

The ideas of Pickstone on knowledge development are suited for linking up with the practical implementation of the social professions. Although this does not apply equally to all professions in the social sector, social professionals are used to reflect on their professional actions.[1] The problem, however, is to make the knowledge and experience that are there during reflection more widely available and to elevate it to a higher design. Experienced professionals may know very well what they must or mustn't do in certain situations, but it is much more difficult for them to indicate what they are exactly doing and why. Their practical knowledge is primarily tacit. The danger of practical knowledge is that, due to its implicit and individual-oriented character, it leads to routine-like actions. Although routines are necessary for professionals in order to tackle complex situations, this should not lead them to exclusively trusting what has worked in the past when faced with a new situation. This would lead to the stagnation of the development of practical knowledge.

The question is how professionals can make their implicit and individual-oriented practical knowledge accessible, as well as deepening and improving it. Answering this question often leads one to refer to concepts such as 'reflective practitioner' and 'communities of practice' as sources of inspiration.

Reflective and Learning Professionals

The idea of the *reflective practitioner* was already introduced by the early 1980s by Donald Schön (1983), but it still generates great interest. Schön exposed the mechanism of how professionals search for suitable solutions to problems in complex and unique practical situations, in which they even have to deal with conflicting values. By reflecting on one's own actions and on strategies, theories, and underlying norms that lie in those actions, professionals can contribute to the development of practical knowledge. In the social sector, Schön's insights are applied mainly to coaching and supervision. This automatically exposes a flaw of the reflective practitioner. To the degree that reflection begins with experiences, it usually starts with the experiences of individual professional practitioners. Reflection should not be limited to individual practitioners however. In addition, the profession and its position in society are under discussion, as is the organisation the professional is part of. The questions are how this knowledge arises via 'lonely' reflection and how it can be made productive for the profession and the organisation.

Communities of Practice (CoPs) offer a partial answer (Wenger 1998; Wenger, McDermott & Snyder 2002; Poell & De Laat 2003; Huysman 2003). Learning and knowledge exchange in a CoP are strongly linked to the everyday learning of professionals and are in the hands of the participants themselves. Those colleagues who share an interest in the same knowledge domains give form to professional deliberations. Together they reflect on events that have taken place during work. Everyday learning at the workplace is thus strengthened. In a CoP, participants explore the 'real' problems and inform each other about the developments in their field. CoPs also risk acquiring a closed character after a while, which would prevent them from exchanging the developed knowledge with professionals in- and outside the organisation. This limits the gains of collective learning. A second disadvantage is that the informal and flexible character of CoPs often makes them invisible to management, which steers mainly formal processes.

Professional Development and Knowledge Development

Concepts like *reflective practitioner* and *communities of practice* offer interesting links for social professionals to contribute to professional development 'from the inside out'. But the danger of biting one's own tail is not unimaginable. For this reason, social professionals must be open to external influences. To this end, co-operation with researchers and scientists is essential. In this context, knowledge development and utilisation should relate not only to formal knowledge via the body of knowledge and skills, but there should also be a focus on the local knowledge and experience-related knowledge of those involved (professionals, volunteers, users). The golden rule reigns among occupational sociologists that the complexity of professional actions is higher as the share of formal knowledge exceeds the share of everyday, practical and tacit knowledge (Freidson 2001). As far as the social professions are concerned, one can detract from this conclusion. Doesn't the ability to combine various sorts of knowledge and sources of knowledge in fact constitute a sign of the complexity of the actions that professionals have to show?

Accordingly, the emphasis must lie not only on the development of formal knowledge via the body of knowledge and skills. A more interesting option is the design of trajectories in which existing practical knowledge is confronted with scientific knowledge, and in which, in turn, new scientific knowledge is tested for its relevance for professional practice. This presumes not only a better unlocking of the already available knowledge, but also – where possible – involving evidence-based practice with practice-based evidence (Van der Laan 2003). This is about searching for meaningful connections between different sorts of data, in which context-specific links are made between scientific insights and locally acquired practical knowledge (Hutschemaekers 2001).

Knowledge Alliances

Social professionals must make alliances with other stakeholders in order to give a greater chance to the development of profession and practice. This requires not only co-operation with scientists and researchers, but also with educators, managers and policymakers. What demands and expectations can be made of the various parties involved?

Professionals

Professionals are expected to constantly bring their own actions up for discussion and establish relations between their own practical knowledge and scientific knowledge, between concrete questions from practice and the results of scientific research. Professionals are also required to actively search for knowledge concerning the effectiveness of methods. To the degree that such knowledge is available, they have to be familiar with it and consider it in their actions (Van Yperen 2003). This is quite different from indiscriminately following eventual guidelines or instructions.

Scientists

Scientists should not claim a monopoly on knowledge, as a strict distinction between knowledge development and professional practice is disastrous for the social professions. As Pickstone shows, it is also not feasible, viewed from an epistemological perspective. Scientists should therefore get professionals more involved in research. In this context,

Kwakman (2003) points to the possible role of knowledge communities, where knowledge developers, disseminators, and users work together to develop more practice-oriented knowledge. In this way, scientists and researchers can reconstruct the actions of practical workers in retrospect, together with those workers. These days, the knowledge and competency of practical workers are not always present at a reflective level and they have to be unlocked. This is a difficult problem for scientists, because in order to do this they have to work within close proximity to practice. They must accurately observe and delve into the capricious dynamics of the actions of professionals, as well as the factors that determine success or failure. Conversely, this presumes that practical workers display the necessary self-respect when it comes to the quality of their own practical knowledge. An important task for scientists, method developers and educators is to formulate 'what we already know', in other words what competent practical workers already use in practice without explicitly formulating it. This line of reasoning leads to an upgrading of practical knowledge from which practical workers can derive the necessary self-respect.

Managers

As an answer to the requirements and enquiries of policymakers, agency managers design, among other things, trajectories for quality care, and try via innovation – even if not scientifically proven – to introduce new ways of working. An essential question is how policymakers, managers and professionals can join forces here. Nowadays, the requirements of policymakers and the responses of managers tend to be burdened by bureaucratic obligations that do not always benefit the quality of the work. When politics and bureaucracy such as patrons and investors determine what should or shouldn't be seen as a socio-societal problem, institutions systematically allow the undermining of their strategic capital, i.e., their connection with the social world of real people. Let us hope that social professionals are better at signalling and identifying developments in the social domain than what comes out of political and managerial negotiations! The fixation upon tested methods and types of work that follow from a specific assignment deserve a counteroffer: the mobilisation of observations and analyses of practical workers.

Educators

Knowledge development deserves more anchoring in the initial formation of social professionals, as well as in competency development after the original study. We have already indicated that in professionals' training there is a strong emphasis on application, in which description and analysis are supposedly more adequate. It is not so much the problems of citizens and politicians that should lead actions, but the problem definition that the profession itself develops, in dialogue with society's interested parties. Increased emphasis on explaining societal issues can make social professionals-in-training more aware of the meaning and scope of their professional actions (analysis). In the initial training period, educators – vocational schools and universities – should pay more attention to what we have called 'primary knowledge development'. The ability to apply specific methods (debt management, mediation) could take shape, for example, in the specialisation, elective programs, or continued education trajectories.

Policymakers

At the moment, policymakers are putting practice under enormous pressure in order for it to work more effectively. They want interventions to be based more on what might work. However, the problem is clearly that the social sector has little scientifically proven knowledge at its disposal. This burdens policymakers with at least two assignments. The first involves doing more research from the policy side. When policymakers want to continue renewal trajectories, they will have to facilitate a lot more research than has been the case up to now. The second assignment relates to the way in which institutions and professionals are made accountable. Policymakers have to leave it up to professionals how to use the available knowledge, even when scientifically proven knowledge is available for certain interventions. The next task for policymakers would be to compare the costs and benefits of the interventions performed with those of other institutions. If the results are lagging far behind, professionals and their institutions should account for it, and attempt to improve their results through development of practice. Learning from colleagues who achieve better results with the same type of clients is an option (Van Yperen 2003: 299). In this way, professionals not only maintain the space to be flexible with situation- and context-specific factors, they are also challenged to look beyond.

The knowledge that is necessary for social professionals to perform in an engaged and efficient manner is available in different places. There is insufficient knowledge exchange. Those involved have the important task of improving the bundling of their efforts in the fields of research, development and innovation, and then offering them to the service of current social issues. It wouldn't hurt professionals, scientists, educators, managers and policymakers to show their willingness to learn more from each other.

Note

1. For example, social workers are more familiar with intervision and supervision than youth workers or community workers (see Spierts et al. 2003).

EMPOWERMENT OF SOCIAL SERVICES PROFESSIONALS

Professional Management of Professionals

Hybrid Organisations and Professional Management in Care and Welfare

Mirko Noordegraaf

Health care and welfare provision have always been complex phenomena – people who tend to be professionals who are caught between private situations, community interests and public values deliver soft services to vulnerable, weak, or powerless individuals. Over time, various types of governance have been introduced in order to organise and provide complex care and welfare. These governance systems have unavoidably been hybrid. Because health care and welfare are service delivery issues; because they involve vulnerable clients and professional providers; and because individual, community and collective interests collide – or conflict – it has proven difficult to leave care and welfare provision exclusively to the state, the market, civil society or individuals. It has always required distinctive combinations of these spheres, especially in small and heterogeneous countries like the Netherlands, which had to introduce intricate, hybrid mechanisms to organise collective action (e. g., Hupe & Meijs 2000).

This does not mean that all of these spheres have always been equally active, or that governance systems have always been balanced. In specific periods, history shows us, specific spheres tended to dominate care and welfare. In previous centuries, the church took an interest in organising services for the sick, the troubled and the poor (e.g., Tuchman 1980). In later periods, municipalities, guilds and wealthy citizens organised or financed service provision (Frijhoff & Spies 1999), due to moral obligations and practical reasons – the wealthy paid for and profited from stable social orders. In the industrial era, private companies took part in health care and welfare settlements, and states became increasingly active. Dutch health care and welfare providers became 'statist' (verstatelijkt) organisations especially during the second half of the 20th century. Embedded within extensive state-based welfare arrangements, they were increasingly financed by public means and therefore controlled through public accountability regimes. These arrangements were bureaucratic as well as professional – in large, bureaucratic organisations, professionalism on the work floor was maintained (see Clarke & Newman 1997).

By the end of the 20th century, state-based welfare settlements were considered too costly, and both market-oriented and businesslike models began to dominate (e.g., Clarke & Newman 1997). In contemporary neo-liberal times, health care and welfare have been subjected to business-like performance regimes (with businesslike managers) and market-oriented control logics. Businesslike models and markets are not the same, and they pull organisations in different directions, but they have much in common, like economic orientations, profit motives, and supply-demand reasoning (Noordegraaf 2004). When both the historical evolution of governance in social sectors and the specificity of social services delivery are taken into account, the economisation and marketisation of care and welfare become controversial phenomena.

Firstly, the motives of businesslike managers and markets to take part in social services delivery lack the moral and practical impetus of earlier private initiatives. In neo-liberal times, motives rest upon cost-control, efficiency and individualistic reasoning, while lacking a sense of the collective. Secondly, states force businesslike managers and markets to become active, pushing social services delivery towards the private spheres but still feeling responsible for the public interest. Consequently, states stick to and extend accountability systems, and ironically use business-like and market logics in the process. Accountability systems have become performance-based planning and control systems. Thirdly, businesslike managers and markets offer certain templates for organising service delivery that are difficult to apply in social services delivery. These templates contain concepts like customers, control and competition, whereas production processes in health care and welfare require concepts like clients (who are much more dependent than customers), professionalism (which is difficult to control) and trust (which is difficult to cultivate in competitive environments). In other words, harming – or destroying – professionalism on the work floor may instead of improving performance actually weaken performance (see also Harrison & Pollitt 1994).

This does not mean that businesslike and market-oriented models are worthless. On the contrary, they will continue to be a part of hybrid governance systems in health care and welfare. In current post-industrial times (e.g., Stehr 1994), financial and cost-control demands are real, and relations between clients and service providers have changed. The decision to either accept or reject managers and markets is pointless. Instead, we should explore how businesslike managers and markets influence each other, as they cannot be aligned easily. We should also explore how they can be combined with professional logics on the work floor and at the street level. This is an organisational challenge that, paradoxically, calls for professional managers. The central question is: how can managers organise health care and welfare in hybrid governance systems that face businesslike and market pressures?

Social Services in Neo-Liberal Societies

Organisations that provide public and social services like care and welfare have become 'trapped'. They must be adapted – or perhaps transformed – so that they can cope with the new demands of post-industrial societies (Stehr 1994). But it is almost impossible to adapt service delivery to new demands in post-industrial societies. First and foremost, the exact nature of these 'new demands' is hard to pin down. We 'know' societies have changed, but how and why remains unclear. The ultimate truth about societal conditions cannot be found, although time and again experts present fresh, absolute truths. The fact that there is no absolute truth may actually be the only truth to be found in contemporary societies.

Contemporary societies are fuzzy societies, with strong yet contradictory stories – dispersed and fragmented truths – about societal change, coming from experts, academics, journalists, politicians and the like. When we take an organisational perspective (assuming organisations still exist), the contradictory nature of new demands becomes much clearer. On the one hand, organisations face an increasing complexity in an era of global networks, multifarious knowledge, acute risks, intangible symbols, uncontrollable incidents, ambivalent citizens, etc. (e.g., Reich 1991; Stehr 1994; Beck 1996; Perrow 2002). On the other hand, organisations – and societies (Ritzer 1993) – face increasing pressures to simplify and 'McDonaldise'. In public services delivery, the latter tendency is fuelled by the 'new public management' movement (Hood 1991; Pollitt & Bouckaert 2000; Noordegraaf 2004) that occurs in 'audit societies' (Power 1999) and 'managerial states' (Clarke & Newman 1997). New public management turns public and social service sectors into businesslike and market-oriented production sectors. Public service organisations are forced to introduce 'planning and control', performance management, measurement systems, quality models, monitoring systems, benchmarking, 'activity-based costing', and so on. Conditions that are hard to comprehend force organisations and managers to act as if they have grasped these conditions. They must set targets, deliver value for money and account for performance. This in itself is contradictory. Service providers introduce businesslike managerial control (cf. Freidson 2001) in order to deliver value for money. They also work on market-oriented consumer control in order to strengthen consumer choice and customer satisfaction. Businesslike managers and markets pull service organisations in different directions.

When we dive into organisational realities, these contradictory forces can cause severe problems. Not just because they pull organisational practices into different directions, but also because they disregard the distinctive nature of production processes in public and social services sectors. Businesslike and market pressures not only contradict each other, they also ignore or negate the professional basis of service provision in sectors like health care and welfare (compare Exworthy & Halford 1999; Freidson 2001). In some ways this is understandable (see, e. g., Exworthy & Halford 1999; Harrison & Pollitt 1994; Harrison 1999). For one thing, professional autonomy is a barrier to organisational cost-control and smooth supply-demand co-ordination, as cost-control and supply-demand arguments are alien to classic professional frames of reference. In addition, professional autonomy and powers are barriers to transparency and accountability, as 'closing' and 'scaling down' tend to accompany strong professional control. It is difficult for clients to hold professionals like medical doctors accountable, so new types of control attempt to de-professionalise, 'proletarianise', bureaucratise, or 'corporatise' professionals (Broadbent et al. 1997; Brock et al. 1999).

At the same time, the provision of services in domains like health care can be said to be unavoidably professional (e.g., Brock et al. 1999). In an empirical sense, social services delivery depends on trained people who treat specific cases by drawing from learned, generic insights. Whether professionalism is defined in a classic sense (e.g., Wilensky 1964; Freidson 2001; Mintzberg 2004) or in a modernised one (e.g., Schön 1983; Brint 1994), such inferential applications of learned, often academic insights can be considered to be the hallmark of professionalism. It is not hard to perceive most public and social services delivery in terms of inferential production processes – service providers at street levels must make informed inferences. Medical doctors treat individual patients with specific histories, symptoms, diseases, and tastes. Medical doctors know a lot, and they must discern what to do when treating individual patients. Welfare workers deal with clients who have distinctive social surroundings, problems and abilities. Effective welfare workers 'know' – have learned to know – how to treat clients, and they also know that some clients cannot really be 'treated'.

Medical and welfare work can thus be routine, but it has many non-routine qualities, or routines can suddenly break down when cases or clients are encountered that are difficult to 'pigeonhole' (cf. Mintzberg 1983). In addition, inferential capacities to treat cases transcend organisations. Professionals need outside training to learn their trade, and professional associations facilitate inferential decision-making. Professional service providers need space to develop their inferential capacities. Inferential behaviour can be standardised, but never completely. Professionals need to see many different cases, for example, so that they can improve comparative insights. They develop 'tacit knowledge' (e.g., Sternberg & Horvath 1999) and need experience to strengthen inferential capacities. Service delivery becomes experiential in particular when complex services are provided, characterised by unclear conditions, contested values, trial-and-error, or latent or long-term effects.

Both inferential and experiential dimensions of public service delivery are at odds with transparent, performance-based, target-driven, 'lean and mean' organising. Inferential and experiential occupational dimensions need to be nurtured in settings, spaces and professional communities that transcend organisational walls. For the new public management movement there is no time to nurture in diffuse settings; organisations must perform, and quickly. For the new public management, customers are all that matters. For professionals, 'service ethics' count (e.g., Wilensky 1964), and service ethics can not be guarded in individualised settings. Although it is not difficult to trace problems – or even perversions – of autonomous professionals, professionals need space and autonomy in order to perform effectively. This includes space to determine what is 'effective'. Because professionals cannot always show directly if and how they are effective, they need space and autonomy in order to institutionalise effective practices.

How can managers guarantee 'effective' social services delivery in unclear settings that require professionals to act inferentially and experientially, as well as force organisations to perform efficiently and transparently?

Professionalising Managers who Deprofessionalise

The fact that professionalism is here to stay is proven by the fact that those who are guilty of managerialising and marketising, and thus weakening professional powers, are themselves professionalising. For a few decades now, executives in health care and welfare organisations have tried to professionalise health care and welfare management. Policy-makers and policy managers at central government levels, who out-rank these managers, try to limit the space that organisational managers and executives can operate in, while they themselves try to professionalise managerial practices. This circularity is ironic. Managers, executives and policy managers who are attempting to control professionalism on the work floor are also trying to professionalise their own trade, and they do so by imitating and emulating classic professionals. They establish professional associations that select, train, develop and supervise professionals. They identify competencies, build educational programs, publish magazines, hold conferences, agree upon codes of conduct and ethical codes, and so on. In terms of classic professionalism, they try to establish a technical base (cf. Wilensky 1964) with standardised knowledge and skills as well as professional ethics (Wilensky 1964; Freidson 2001), both of which are guarded by state-guaranteed jurisdictions (Abbott 1988).

The fact that managers and executives have started professionalising could be expected. Decades ago, Wilensky (1964) even wondered whether we were starting to witness the 'professionalisation of everyone' in post-industrial times. No wonder, when we recognise the fact that 'knowledge workers' in post-industrial or knowledge societies work with information and knowledge, which they apply to specific cases, instances and situations, just like medical doctors. Managers and executives are prominent examples of such knowledge workers. In addition, the neo-liberal attack on the welfare state and the public sector was an attack on professional powers, so managers and executives had to develop counter-vailing powers – which they found in models for professional powers of medical doctors, lawyers and the like. The attack led to the de-professio-nalisation of professionals in health care, welfare and other social do-mains, and paradoxically fuelled a professionalisation of managers and executives in health care and welfare. The neo-liberal attack also deter-mined the content of managerial and executive professionalism. To manage professionally in fields like health care implies a businesslike and market-oriented approach. Health care organisations have to be-come normal, integrated companies (e.g., Kruithof 2005) that are guided by market or quasi-market factors for health care provision (see also Le-Grand & Bartlett 1994). They have to deliver products to customers, with optimal value for money and returns on investment, by way of efficient, co-ordinated, and accountable production processes (see also Meurs & Van der Grinten 2005). This required executives and managers who must control health care professionals (see, e.g., Harrison & Pollitt 1994), and various mechanisms have been instrumental in this process:

- Planning and control cycles include targets, contracts, results and accountability. Professionals must stick to production agreements.
- Divisional management, with organisational divisions, is governed strategically by executive boards. Professionals must contribute to divisional performance.
- Quality control, through peer review procedures, or using quality models such as the EFQM model (www.efqm.org; www.ink.nl).
- Performance measurement, with monitoring and benchmarking, using tools such as 'dashboards' and 'thermometers'. Professional behaviour is measured.
- Evidence-based medicine, with transparent medical work that has been proven to work and be effective.
- Medical managers, who are both medical doctors and managers at the same time. They manage doctors and nurses.
- Salaried professionals, instead of 'free' professionals. Professionals like doctors are turned into regular employees.

Professional Managers and Executives

Whether managers and executives can become professionals is and will remain a contested issue. According to some, it is possible (Brock et al. 1999), according to others, professional managers are a logical impossi-bility (Raelin 1986; Mintzberg 2004). Irrespective of these theoretical debates, managers and executives are professionalising – they have started to see themselves as professionals, they use words like 'professional', and they have started to introduce and institutionalise traditional professional models in order to get a grip on managerial practices. A broad trend towards professionalising managers can be witnessed, in both public and private domains, accompanied by a professionalisation industry, with advisors, conferences, books, documents, models, etc. Health care managers and executives are one of the best examples of attempts to 'create' professional managers, by way of (e.g., Noordegraaf & Meurs 2002):

- Professional associations, such as the Dutch association of health care executives (NVZD) that regulate executive work (www.nvzd.nl).
- Magazines, such as the Dutch ZM Magazine, read by most health care executives and managers.
- Evidence-based management (EBM), as a counterweight to evidence-based medicine, with competencies and behaviours that have proven to be effective.
- Protocols, agreements about aspects of executive or managerial work, e.g., regarding executive salaries and bonuses.
- Codes of conduct, professional agreements that identify and formalise appropriate behaviour.
- Schooling and training, such as master classes and Master of Public Health Courses, organised by universities (e.g., www.bmg.eur.nl).
- Management trainee and high potential programs, in order to stimulate management development.

As far as the Dutch Association of Health Care Executives (NVZD) is concerned, its 'strategy' is framed in terms of professionalism. It is circumscribed as follows (www.nvzd.nl):

> The NVZD is the special interest group of health care executives. The NVZD promotes professional practices and represents their interests.

In other domains, like welfare and social work, comparable attempts can be traced, but compared with health care they are relatively weak attempts at enhancing managerial professionalism. This is explained firstly by social work and welfare not being characterised by strong professionals on the work floor, and secondly by the fact that welfare organisations used to differ – on average – from health care organisations in terms of size, financial capacities, technology, and relative autonomy from (local) government. Nevertheless, we see comparable patterns. In social work and welfare, professional managers and executives are created by such mechanisms as:

- Associations, like the Dutch MO Group or Social Entrepreneurs Group (www.mogroep.nl).
- Magazines, ranging from brochures and reports with, e.g., standard contracts to journals with quick, useful, and necessary information.

- Research and knowledge, like scenario studies that portray welfare and social work 10 or 15 years from now.
- Schooling and training programs, such as university- and polytechnic-based Masters degrees in social policy and social work in urban areas (e.g., www.uva.nl).

The Dutch MO Group, which brings together most of the welfare and social work organisations, literally states (see www.mogroep.nl):

> Social services providers are professional. They take responsibility and ask others to do the same: health care providers, decision makers, officials, educators, citizens and their environments. They know that society offers opportunities for organisations and individuals. They are sources of commitment.

This is not the end of the story. Executives and managers in charge of services delivery are not the only ones who have started professionalising. High-ranking government policymakers who feel responsible and are held accountable for governing policy fields like health care and welfare have also started to see themselves as professional public managers. Policy managers at central bodies like the Ministry of Health and Welfare have initiated health care and welfare reform, and have turned de-professionalisation of real professionals on the work floor into law – less powerful doctors, more powerful executives – at the same time resisting powerful executives. This is evidenced by attempts to weaken entrepreneurial initiatives in or around health care organisations, which resulted from more autonomous, professional executive behaviour. It is also evidenced by more general policy attempts to control health care systems. Health care executives must introduce large-scale nationwide regimes, like 'diagnosis-related treatment' systems, and must compete on a quasi-market level within strict public and regulatory frameworks that are being introduced in order to create and maintain 'level playing fields'. In social work and welfare, plans for a new law – the Social Support Act (WMO) – have produced a grand design for social services, with decentralised and privatised service delivery. This law grants freedoms to local organisations and service providers, but also limits freedoms, e.g., through new standards, contracts and performance requirements.

These policy managers – another irony – are trying to become professional policy managers, while imitating the classic professions. They establish technical bases with knowledge, skills and competencies, and try to establish professional associations in order to institutionalise professional control. The central governments of numerous countries have, in particular, witnessed the rise of a new managerial class, the 'senior public service' (SPS). In Dutch central government, the following mechanisms have been introduced:

- Associations, like the Dutch SPS (ABD, www.algemenebestuurs-dienst.nl) for all upper-level public managers in central government (900 managers).
- Competency profiles, like the ABD competency profile, with seven core competencies (the 'magnificent seven'), and 35 additional competencies.
- Mobility programs, so that organisational pillars are torn down and (central) government works as one.
- Publications, like ABD publications, magazines and journals, e.g., the Dutch (now defunct) magazine Publiek management, and books on leadership.
- Platforms, like conferences and meetings, such as Dutch Top Management Team Meetings.
- Schooling and training programs for managers, like the Candidates Program for upcoming ABD managers.
- Codes of conduct, for instance codes for responsible or ethical behaviour, or for remuneration.

Professional Managing in Service Delivery

The foregoing must not be exaggerated, as it sketches a picture that is rather formal and too black-and-white. The rough sketch of de-professionalising or proletarianising experts on the one hand, and professionalising managers and executives on the other, presents a simple, unrealistic zero-sum analysis. In daily reality, experts and specialists on the work floor are and remain relatively autonomous and powerful professionals, especially in health care, and managers and executives have not always become strong organisational players. Paradoxically, moves towards 'integrated' companies in health care have gone hand in hand with the strengthening of professional bodies and negotiating positions within hospitals (Kruithof 2005). The interplay between experts and executives might also lead to win-win outcomes, especially when those working at the service levels fight against outside forces like central government. In addition, professionalising policy managers who create new governance systems and who make managerial laws – driven by ideas about efficiency, cost-control and quality – do not automatically limit space and powers at the service levels. Health care executives, for instance, have plenty of possibilities to establish distinctive service realities, not despite but thanks to a bewildering array of laws, regulations and requirements.

Mild forms of exaggeration might be necessary, however, to put the current state of affairs into perspective. Too many complaints can be heard in dismissing critical analyses of developments in health care and welfare as nonsensical. In many respects, health care and welfare are heading in the wrong direction. This does not mean that managers are to blame, as is frequently assumed (e.g., Tonkens 2003; Van de Brink et al. 2005). Professionals are also to blame – if blame is necessary. Classic professionals who are primarily loyal to professional communities cannot avoid new loyalties to organisational surroundings. They can not negate blurred financial and client realities, so they have to become 'organisational professionals' or 'expert professionals' (Brint 1994; also, Brock et al. 1999) who combine professional patient care with matters of organisational capacity and client choice. New discourses are thus needed which deconstruct simple 'manager versus professional' dichotomies, and which show how managers and executives can combine organisational responsibilities with social, public and political outlooks, and embrace a sense of the collective. Professionalism on the work floor and at managerial levels must be perceived as a hybrid phenomenon. A hybridised professionalism instead of a pure one suits today's unclear realities. If executives and managers have distinctive responsibilities for organising health care and welfare because it is their formal duty, legal assignment and socially perceived calling, then the following question is, how can they professionally organise and manage in health care and welfare?

One thing is clear by now – professional managers can neither strive towards maintaining loose organisations of professionals nor towards establishing simple businesslike organisations. This awareness has led to pleas for optimising 'professional organisations' that combine the best of both worlds (Brock et al. 1999). Professionalism on the work floor is simultaneously respected and restrained via all sorts of means and mechanisms. Means like flexible organisational structures, decentralised organisational models, shared responsibilities, professional cultures, and knowledge management are used to that end. These insights are valuable, as they express an emphasis on hybrid organisations, but they are also insufficient. Given that organisations are not static entities and require continuous organising (Weick 1995), the question is, how can managers organise and maintain professional organisations? This is a matter of day-to-day behaviour, of talk, text and action, of conversational behaviour (Kaufman 1980; Brunsson 1985; Alvesson 1996; Noordegraaf 2000), which takes place in specific organisational surroundings and 'streams' (see also Langley et al. 1995) that are full of loosely defined and ambiguous issues. Professional organising and managing requires an understanding of how practitioners make sense of daily realities – also by way of grand concepts, like 'professional organisation' – and of how they enact organisational realities and act in such realities. What do professional organisations mean? How do executives and managers establish professional organisations? What do managers actually do to enact them? On the basis of earlier research in public (service) domains, including empirical studies in public service delivery (e.g., LeGrand & Bartlett 1994; Exworthy & Halford 1999; Grit & Meurs 2005) and more anecdotal stories (e.g., Idenburg 1999), the following features can be said to characterise professional managers in public service delivery:

Public Service Managers are Institutionalists

When organised realities are portrayed as local and conversational but are embedded within broader institutional frameworks like laws, regulations, routines, educational programs, ideologies and symbols, managerial behaviour is perceived to be institutionally embedded (see, e.g., March & Olsen 1989; Scott 1995). This means that individual behaviour in domains like health care and welfare must be linked to shared ways of doing, thinking, and feeling that have developed and evolved over time. Health care, for instance, contains institutionalised ideas about services, illness, expertise and patients, and institutionalised ideologies that emphasise aspects like care, solidarity and needs. These ideas and ideologies, which express themselves through laws, professional ethics, codes, vocabularies and practices, are difficult to change. Empirically, they provide barriers to change; normatively, they provide shields against grand-scale and potentially dangerous interventions (Scott 1998). Businesslike and market-oriented models ignore institutional surroundings, and this alone creates problems. Other problems also arise, as institutionalised features also embody values (Selznick 1984), which are placed at risk. As long as we perceive health care, collectively, as curing and caring for patients, these values should be upheld. This means that managing and organising production and services delivery will never be like normal production in private spheres. It will inevitably be characterised by asymmetric relations between providers and clients, contradictory private, social and public interests, and contested measures of effectiveness and success. In short, care and welfare production will be irregular, and professional managers are aware of this. They balance change and conservation (Terry 1996), and seek transformations that are in tune with the features and logic of production practices. In practical terms this means, inter alia, that managers and executives should manage things hands-on instead of hands-off (Sayles 1989), be visible and walk around (Peters & Austin 1985), have a 'feel' for domains, and understand the stories, histories and idiosyncrasies.

Public Service Managers are Standardisers

All organised action, especially on a large scale, requires co-ordination, and most co-ordination calls for standards. Professionalism can be seen as a specific means for co-ordinating organised action: by standardising skills and values, protected and regulated by professional bodies, professionals know what to do (cf. Mintzberg 1983). Businesslike and market-oriented management negates this – it attempts to standardise work processes (e.g., planning and control, quality models) as well as outputs (e. g., contracts, accountability). This will eventually cause trouble, especially when applied to professional management. Most importantly, standardised work processes and outputs assume that goals, objectives, and problems are given, and that managers can decide how to reach objectives and solve problems. The goal of managerial action, however, could also be to discover goals. Besides, the problem in organisational realities often is: what is the problem? Organisational realities are ambiguous; interpretations of what has happened, what can and should be done, and who has to be involved, differ (e.g., Weick 1995). In other words, managers and executives will not work within available standards – they set standards, and standard setting is a continuous, subtle process (e.g., Brunsson & Jacobsen 2000). Such standards are construed, developed and set in subtle daily talks, interactions and texts. From a practical perspective this means that managers are able to use meetings and papers for setting standards (Noordegraaf 2000), play with conflicting standards (Brunsson & Adler 1989), establish appropriate rules, routines and rituals, and respect and guard (professional) standards.

Public Service Managers are Politicians

Local practices are part of institutionalised domains; standards come from and affect outside surroundings. Professional managers do not conform directly to these surroundings however. Situations differ, and professional managers show tendencies to act as 'associated rivals' (cf. Dogan 2003): they associate themselves with managerial communities, but other managers are rivals too. They might be rivals in the sense of being competitors when managerial positions become vacant, fighting for money, having different opinions on appropriate courses of action, having different stakes in terms of who they want to serve, or holding different positions on 'rankings' that are made public in newspapers or through the Internet. Because neo-liberal times are characterised by capacity problems, financial scarcity, strategic ambiguities, emancipated clients and public pressures to be accountable, such rivalries have become rather normal. To get a businesslike grip on such complexities and to normalise conditions can be considered as being abnormal. Health care and welfare management has moral and political twists. Executives and managers will have to find ways to act responsibly, make choices and weigh the options (Grit & Meurs 2005). Executives and managers are drawn into politics, with activities like priority-setting, as capacities are limited (e.g., Hunter 1997; see also Fisher 1998), accounting, as performances must be accounted for but are hard to account for (Noordegraaf & Abma 2003), and legitimising, as trust in public services has declined. Executives and managers must, for example, determine how to deal with uninsured illegal foreigners who need care, which clients are eligible for quicker treatment when several clients need to be treated, whether to treat citizens from ethnic minorities abroad when they go back to their home countries for summer vacation, if they should spend money on cases that barely can be treated, etc. In practical terms, this means executives and managers are visible, are open about choices, challenge themselves, introduce checks and balances, confront dilemmas (Grit & Meurs 2005), account for their actions and act courageously, also vis-à-vis politicians (also Meurs & Van der Grinten 2005).

Conclusion

The foregoing can be summarised in a few simple argumentative steps. Domains like care and welfare are hybrid and call for hybrid governance. Hybrid governance calls for subtle mechanisms that meet private, social and public interests, and it calls for professional managers, who practise hybridised forms of professionalism. In neo-liberal times, however, it is difficult to uphold hybrid mechanisms and means. Market and business models dominate; organisations are pressured to act in a businesslike and market-oriented fashion. This has started to colour managerial professionalism: Executives and managers have not only started to imitate classic professionals, like medical doctors, in order to limit powers of classic professionals, but they have also started to embed experts on the work floor in the areas of problematic planning and control and performance regimes. Ironically, this does not improve but actually harms organisational performance. Merely blaming managers is nonsensical, and notions like 'professional organisations' are insufficient to compensate for these worrisome tendencies. Executives and managers in the blurred fields of care and welfare need to find ways of professional organisation and management. Professional executives and managers in service domains like health care and welfare can be said to be standardisers who are aware of the politics of public organising, and set standards that are in tune with local institutionalised surroundings. Professional managers are critical of popular models, transgress simple dichotomies – and professional experts do the same.

N/A↩

About the contributors

Sophie Body-Gendrot is Professor at the Sorbonne University in Paris. Her research focuses on the comparison of neighbourhoods, violence and immigrants. One of her latest books include *The social control of cities* (1998).

Celia Davies is a sociologist and Visiting Professor at the Nursing Research Unit, King's College London. She was formerly Professor of Health Care at the Open University, Milton Keynes, UK. Her most recent book (with Margie Wetherell and Elizabeth Barnett), *Citizens at the Centre: deliberative participation in healthcare decisions*, will be published in late 2006.

Jan Willem Duyvendak is Professor of Sociology at the University of Amsterdam, the Netherlands. His main interests are social movements, city policies (more in particular on the link between physical and social development) integration topics, citizenship and labour & care issues.

Jeroen Gradener is cultural psychologist and lecturer at the AVANS Academy of Social Studies (Breda/Den Bosch), the Netherlands. At the Academy, he is chairman of the Research Community 'Macro Social Work'. His fields of interests are Community Organisation and Social Entrepreneurship.

Giel Hutschemaekers is Professor of Professionalisation of Care at the Radboud University Nijmegen and director of the Gelderse Roos Institute for Professionalisation, the Netherlands. He has been (co)author of several publications about the organisation of (mental) health care and professionals who work in this area. His main research interest at this moment is the empowerment of professionals as well as clients.

Trudie Knijn is Professor of Interdisciplinary Social Science and member of the Interuniversity Center for Social Science Theory and Methodology, Utrecht University, the Netherlands. Her main areas of work are comparative welfare state studies and social policy. She is particularly interested in transformations in professional and informal care, and in family policy and family relations. Recently she published with Ute Gerhard and Anja Weckwert *Working Mothers in Europe. A Comparison of Policies and Practices*, 2005, Cheltenham: Edward Elgar Publishers.

Monique Kremer is research fellow at the Netherlands Scientific Council for Government Policy. Her research interests include care, citizenship and the welfare state in a European comparative perspective. She has recently co-edited (with Menno Hurenkamp) *Vrijheid verplicht*, on the limits of the policy concept of free choice (2005).

Maarten Loopmans works at the Institute for Social and Economic Geography of the University of Leuven (Belgium). His research focuses on neighbourhood social networks, public space, active citizenship and urban policy.

Mirko Noordegraaf works at the Utrecht School of Governance (USG) of Utrecht University, The Netherlands, as an associate professor. He focuses on organisation and management themes in the public sphere, with specific emphasis on the work and behaviour of public managers. At this moment he heads the research project "Professionalism in Public Domains", in which the professionalization of public managers is explored.

Peter Selten is a lecturer at the Department of Interdisciplinary Social Sciences at Utrecht University, the Netherlands. His research interests include youth, youth culture and family care.

Marcel Spierts is a lecturer and researcher at the School for Social Work of the Hogeschool van Amsterdam, the Netherlands. He has published and (co)edited several books on professionalism in the field of social work and community development – including *Werken aan Openheid en Samenhang* (2000) and *Beroep in Ontwikkeling* (1998).

Bea Tiemens is senior investigator at the Gelderse Roos, Institute for Professionalisation, the Netherlands. She has been (co)-author of several publications about management of mental health problems in primary care.

Evelien Tonkens is Professor of Active Citizenship at the Department of Sociology and Anthropology at the University of Amsterdam. She is also editor of *TSS, Tijdschrift voor Sociale Vraagstukken* and columnist for the daily Dutch newspaper *de Volkskrant*. Her articles and books deal with changes in ideals and practices of citizenship in relation to changes in professional practices and other aspects of welfare state revision.

Margo Trappenburg is a political scientist employed at the Utrecht School of Governance (Utrecht University) and Professor of Patient perspectives at the Erasmus University (Rotterdam, the Netherlands). Her research interests include modern political philosophy, professionalism and democracy in the health care system. She published in *Health Care Analysis* and in the *Journal of Political Philosophy*.

Justus Uitermark was trained as a human geographer and is currently attached to the Amsterdam School for Social Science Research, University of Amsterdam. His main interest is in urban sociology and urban policy. He recently published *De sociale controle van achterstandswijken*.

Marleen van der Haar is a cultural anthropologist preparing her PhD dissertation at the Utrecht School of Governance, Utrecht University, the Netherlands. Her research project focuses on social workers and diversity in the multicultural society.

Werner Vogd is a cultural anthropologist and sociologist, employed at the Free University of Berlin, Germany. His research topics include professionalisation, organizational sociology, qualitative methods and system theory.

References

Abbott, A. (1988). *The System of Professions: An Essay on the Division of Expert Labor*. Chicago and London: University of Chicago Press.

Achterhuis, H. (1979). *De markt van welzijn en geluk*. Baarn: Ambo.

Allen, J. (2003). *Lost Geographies of Power*. Oxford: Blackwell.

Allsop, J. (2002). 'Regulation and the Medical Profession'. In Allsop, J. and M. Saks (eds.). *Regulating the Health Professions*. London: Sage.

Allsop, J. and Mulcahy, L. (1998). 'Maintaining Professional Identity: Doctors' Responses to Complaints'. *Sociology of Health and Illness* 20, 6: 812-34.

Alvesson, M. (1996). *Communication, Power and Organization*. Berlin: De Gruyter.

Anis, M. (2005). 'Talking about Culture in Social Work Encounters: Immigrant Families and Child Welfare in Finland', *European Journal of Social Work*, 8 (1), 3-19.

Antwerpenaar, De (2005). 'Opsinjoren maakt van bewoners weer buren [Opsinjoren makes residents into neighbours]'. *De Antwerpenaar*, 3 (48), 12.

Appleby, J. and A. Coote. (2002). *Five Year Health Check: a review of government health policy 1997-2002*. London: King's Fund.

Arts, S. (2002). *Caring as an Occupation: Content and Quality of Working Life among Home Helps*. Utrecht: Nivel.Baerveldt, C. (1999). *Culture and the Consensual Coördination of Actions*. Ph.D. diss., Radboud University Nijmegen.

Baerveldt, C. (1999). *Culture and the Consensual Coordination of Actions*. Ph.D. diss., Radboud University Nijmegen.

Baggott, R. J. Allsop, K. and Jones. (2004). *Speaking Out for Patients and Careers*. London: Palgrave.

Banks, S. (2004). *Ethics, Accountability and the Social Professions*. London: Palgrave Macmillan.

Barnes, M. (1997). *Care, Communities and Citizens*. London: Longman.

Bauman, Z. (2000). *Liquid Modernity*. Cambridge: Polity Press.

Bauman, Z. (2001). 'The Great War of Recognition'. *Theory, Culture and Society* 18, 2-3, 137-150.

Baumann, G. (1999). *The Multicultural Riddle: Rethinking National, Ethnic and Religious Identities*. New York: Routledge.

Beck, U. (1992). *Risk Society: Towards a New Modernity*, London: Sage.

Beer, P.T. de (2001). *Over werken in de post-industriële samenleving*. Ph.D. dissertation, The Hague: UvA, SCP.

Benhabib, S. (2002). *The Claims of Culture: Equality and Diversity in the Global Era*. Princeton: Princeton University Press.

Berg, J.Th.J. van den and H.A.A. Molleman (1977). *Crisis in de Nederlandse politiek* 2nd ed. Alphen a/d Rijn: Samsom.

Berg, M. (1996). 'Practices of Reading and Writing: The Constitutive Role of the Patient Record in Medical Work'. *Sociology of Health and Illness*, 18 (4), 499-524.

Berg, M., R.T. Meulen and M. van den Burg (2001). 'Guidelines for Appropriate Care: The Importance of Empirical Normative Analysis'. *Health Care Analysis*, 9, 77-99.

Black, N. and E. Thompson (1993). 'Obstacles to Medical Audit: British Doctors Speak Out'. *Social Science and Medicine* 36, 7, 849-856.

Blanchard, Ch.G., M.S. Labrecque, J.C. Ruckdeschel, J. and E.B. Blanchard (1988). 'Information and Decision-Making Preferences of Hospitalized Adult Cancer Patients'. *Social Science and Medicine*, 27 (11), 1139-1145.

Blank, R.H. and V. Burau (2004). *Comparative Health Policy*. Macmillan: Palgrave.

Blok, G. (2004). *Baas in eigen brein. Antipsychiatrie in Nederland 1965-1985*. Amsterdam: Nieuwezijds.

Blommaert, J. and C. Bulcaen (2000). 'Critical Discourse Analysis', *Annual Review of Anthropology*, 29, 447-466.

Body-Gendrot, S. (1993). *Ville et violence. L'irruption de nouveaux acteurs*. Paris: Presses Universitaires de France.

Body-Gendrot, S. (2000). *The Social Control of Cities? A Comparative Perspective*. Oxford: Blackwell.

Body-Gendrot, S. (2002). 'The Dangerous Others: Changing Views on Urban Risks and Violence in France'. In Eade J. and C. Mele (eds.) *Understanding the City: Contemporary and Future Perspectives*. Oxford: Blackwell, pp. 82-106.

Body-Gendrot, S. (2003). 'Local Governance, Community Organization, and Crime: The Case of France'. In S. Body-Gendrot and M. Gittell (eds.), *Social Capital and Social Citizenship*. Lanham: Lexington, pp. 25-51.

Body-Gendrot, S. (2005). (forthcoming). 'France. The Politicization of Youth Justice'. In J. Muncie and B. Goldson (eds.) *Comparative Youth Justice*. London: Sage.

Body-Gendrot, S. (2006, forthcoming). 'France. The Politicization of Youth Justice'. In J. Muncie and B. Goldson (eds.) *Comparative Youth Justice*. London: Sage.

Body-Gendrot, S. and C. Withold de Wenden (2003). *Police et discriminations raciales : le tabou français*. Paris: Editions de l'atelier.

Boer, N. de, and J.W. Duyvendak (2004). Welzijn. In H.Dijstelbloem, P.L. Meurs and E.K. Schrijvers, *Maatschappelijke dienstverlening. Een onderzoek naar vijf sectoren* (WRR Verkenningen nr. 6). Amsterdam: Amsterdam University Press.

Bouma, J. and E. Brandt (2005). Farma-industrie krijgt patiëntenclubs in greep; het geld en de pillen, in: *Trouw*, 5-2, p. V2.

Bourdieu, P. (1997). *Méditations pascaliennes*. Paris: Seuil.

Bourdieu, P. (1998). 'The Left Hand and the Right Hand of the State' interview with R.P. Droit and T. Ferenczi. In *Acts of Resistance: Against the New Myths of Our Time*. Cambridge: Polity Press.

Bourdieu, P. et al. (2002). *The Weight of the World: Social Suffering in Contemporary Society*. Cambridge: Polity Press.

Bovens, M. (2003). 'Zelfstandigheid tussen markt en meten'. In: *Tijdschrift voor de Sociale Sector* 57, 10, 14-15.

Bovens, M. and P. 't Hart (2005). 'Publieke verantwoording: zegen en vloek'. In W. Bakker and K. Yesilkagit (eds.) *Publieke verantwoording*. Amsterdam: Boom, pp. 245-264.

Braga, A. and C. Winship (2006 forthcoming). 'Partnership, Accountability, and Innovation: Clarifying Boston's Experience with Pulling Levers'. In *Comparative Perspectives on Legitimacy and the Criminal Justice System*. R. Sampson, Ch. Windship, T. Tyler, J. Fagan and A. Braga (eds.) New York: Russell Sage.

Brink, G. van den (2002). *Mondiger of moeilijker? Een studie naar de politieke habitus van hedendaagse burgers*. The Hague: Scientific Council for Government Policy.

Brink, G. van den (2004). *Schets van een beschavingsoffensief. Over normen, normaliteit en normalisatie in Nederland* (WRR Verkenning 3). Amsterdam and Den Haag: Amsterdam University Press.

Brink, G. van den, Th. Jansen and D. Pessers (eds.) (2005). *Beroepszeer*. Amsterdam: Boom.

Brint, S. (1994). *In an Age of Experts: the Changing Role of Professionals in Politics and Public Life*. Princeton, N.J.: Princeton University Press

Broadbent, M.D. et al. (1997). *The End of the Professions?* London: Routledge.

Brock, D., M. Powell and C.R. Hinings (eds.) (1999). *Restructuring the Professional Organisation*. London: Routledge.

Brown, Ph. and S. Zavestoski (eds.) (2005). *Social Movements in Health*. Oxford: Blackwell.

Bruce, T. and W.C. Sanderson (eds.) (2005). *Evidence-Based Psychosocial Practices: Past, Present and Future*. Hoboken: John Wiley & Sons.

Bruijn, H. de (2001). *Prestatiemeting in de publieke sector. Tussen professie en verantwoording*. Utrecht: Lemma.

Brunsson, N. (1985). *The Irrational Organisation*. Chichester: John Wiley.

Brunsson, N. and N.J. Adler (1989). *The Organization of Hypocrisy*. Chichester: John Wiley.

Brunsson, N. and B. Jacobsen (2000). *A World of Standards*. Oxford: Oxford University Press.

Bulcaen, C. and J. Blommaert (1999). 'De constructie van 'klassieke gevallen. Case management in de interculturele hulpverlening'. In F. Glastra (ed.), *Organisaties en diversiteit. Naar een contextuele benadering van intercultureel management*. Utrecht: Lemma, pp. 139-158.

Campbell, C. and S. Jovcelovitch (2000). Health, Community and Development: Towards a Social Psychology of Participation. *Journal of Community & Applied Social Psychology* 10(4), 255-270.

Carr-Saunders, A.M. and P. A. Wilson (1933). *The Professions*. Oxford: Clarendon Press.

Casparie, A.F. et al. (2001). *Evaluatie kwaliteitswet zorginstellingen*. The Hague: ZonMW.

Cawston, P.G. and R.S. Barbour (2003). 'Clients or Citizens? Some Consideration for Primary Care Organisations'. *British Journal of General Practice*, Sept. 2003, 716-722.

CBS (Centraal Bureau voor de Statistiek) (2002). *Maandstatistiek van de bevolking*. Jaargang 50 – juli 2002, Voorburg and Heerlen: CBS.

CBS (Centraal Bureau voor de Statistiek) (2004). *Allochtonen in Nederland 2004*. Voorburg: CBS.

Chamberlayne P. and P. Sudbury (2001). Editorial. *Journal of Social Work Practice* 15, 2, 125-130.

Chamberlayne, P., J. Bornat and U. Apitzsch (2004). *Biographical Methods and Professional Practice*. Bristol: Policy Press.

Charles, C., A. Gafni and T. Whelan (1999). 'Decision-Making in the Physician-Patient Encounter: Revisiting the Shared Treatment Decision-Making Model'. *Social Science and Medicine*, 49, 651-661.

Choquet, M. (2000). 'La violence des jeunes: données épidémiologiques'. In C. Rey (ed.) *Les Adolescents face à la violence*. Paris: Syros, 61-74.

Clarke, J. (1998). 'Doing the Right Thing? Managerialism and Social Welfare'. In P. Abbott and L. Meerabeau, *The Sociology of the Caring Professions*. London and Philadelphia: UCL Press, Taylor & Francis Group.

Clarke, J. (2003). *Performing for the Public: Evaluation, Evidence and Evangelism in Social Policy*, a paper prepared for the Social Policy Association Conference, University of Teesside, July 2003.

Clarke, J. and J. Newman (1997). *The Managerial State: Power, Politics and Ideology in the Remaking of Social Welfare*. London: Sage.

Cochrane, A.L. (1972). *Effectiveness and Efficiency. Random Reflections on Health Services*. Cambridge: Cambridge University Press.

Conlon, E. (2004). *Blue Blood*. New York: Riverhead.

Conseil de l'Europe (1994). *Formation de la police concernant les relations avec les migrants et les groupes ethniques. Directives pratiques*. Strasbourg: Les Editions du Conseil de l'Europe.

Cornwall, A and J. Gaventa (2001). *From Users and Choosers to Makers and Shapers: Repositioning Participation in Social Policy*. IDS-working paper, Brighton (www.ids.ac.uk/publications).

Coulter, A. (2002). *The Autonomous Patient*. London: Nuffield Trust.

Coulter, A. (2003). 'An Unacknowledged Workforce: Patients as Partners in Healthcare'. In Davies, C. *The Future Health Workforce*. Basingstoke: Macmillan.

Cox, K., D. de Louw, J. Verhoef and C. Kuiper (2004). *Evidence based practice voor verpleegkundigen. Methodiek en implementatie*. Utrecht: Lemma.

Cruikshank, B. (1999). *The Will to Empower: Democratic Citizens and Other Subjects*. New York: Cornell University Press.

Dahrendorf, R. (2004). 'Succes van diensten niet meetbaar'. *de Volkskrant*, 19 januari 2004: 7

Dalrymple, Th. (2001). *Life at the Bottom: The Worldview that Makes the Underclass*. London: Ivan R. Dee.

Davies, C. (1995). *Gender and the Professional Predicament in Nursing*. Buckingham: Open University Press.

Davies, C. (2000). 'Improving the Quality of Services'. In A. Brechin, H. Brownand, M.A. Eby (eds.). *Critical Practice in Health and Social Care*. London: Sage.

Davies, C. (ed.) (2003). *The Future Health Workforce*. Basingstoke: Macmillan.

Davies, C. and A. Beach (2000). *Interpreting Professional Self-Regulation: A History of the United Kingdom Central Council for Nursing, Midwifery and Health Visiting*. London: Routledge.

Dawson, M. (1994). *Behind the Mule*. Princeton: Princeton University Press.

Deber, R.B., N., Kraetschmer and J. Irvine (1996). 'What Role Do Patients Wish to Play in Treatment Decision Making?' *Archives Internal Medicine*, 156 (13), 1414-1420.

Decker, P. De, C. Kesteloot, F. De Maesschalck and J. Vranken (2005). 'Revitalizing the City in an Anti-Urban Context: Extreme Right and the Rise of Urban Policies in Flanders, Belgium'. *International Journal of Urban and Regional Research*, 29 (1) 152-171.

Department of Health (1997). *The New NHS. Modern. Dependable.* CM3807, London: Stationery Office.

Department of Health (1998). *A First Class Service: Quality in the New NHS – a consultation paper*. London: Department of Health.

Department of Health (1999). *Supporting Doctors, Protecting Patients: a consultation paper*. London: Department of Health.

Department of Health (2000a). *A Health Service of All the Talents: Developing the NHS Workforce. Consultation document on the review of workforce planning*. London: Department of Health.

Department of Health (2000b). *The NHS Plan. A plan for investment. A plan for reform*. London: Department of Health.

Department of Health (2002). *Changing Workforce Programme. New ways of working in health care*, London: Department of Health.

DGV (Nederlands Instituut voor verantwoord medicijngebruik) (2005). Sponsoring van patiëntenorganisaties door de farmaceutische industrie. Onderzoeksverslag. Utrecht: DGV.

Dibben, P. and P. Higgins (2004). 'NPM: Marketisation, Managerialism and Consumerism'. In P. Dibben, G. Wood and T. Roper (eds.) *Contesting Public Sector Reforms. Critical Perspectives, International Debates*. Houndmills: Palgrave, pp. 26-37.

Diekstra, R.F.W., M. van Toor, M. den Ouden and M. Schweitzer (2002). *Vriendelijker, verantwoordelijker, veiliger. Stadsetiquette: van idee naar programma*. Rotterdam: Gemeente Rotterdam.

Dijk, R. van and E. van Dongen (2000). 'Migrants and Mental Health Care in the Netherlands'. In P. Vulpiani, J. M. Comelles and E. van Dongen (eds.), *Health for all, all in Health: European Experiences on Health Care for Migrants*. Perugia: Cidis/Alisei, pp. 47-68.

Dillon, A. (2001). NICE and Clinical Governance'. In M. Lugon and J. Secker-Walker (eds.) *Advancing Clinical Governance*. London: Royal Society of Medicine Press.

Dogan, M. (2003). 'Is There a Ruling Class in France?' *Comparative Sociology*, 2 (1), 17-89.

Doorn, J.A.A. and C.J.M. Schuyt (ed.) (1978). *De stagnerende verzorgingsstaat*. Meppel: Boom.

Durkheim, E. (1957). *Professional Ethics and Civic Morals*. London: Routledge and Kegan Paul.

Duyvendak, J.W. (1997). *Waar blijft de politiek? Essays over paarse politiek, maatschappelijk middenveld en sociale cohesie*. Amsterdam: Boom.

Duyvendak, J.W. (1999). *De planning van de ontplooiing: wetenschap, politiek en de maakbare samenleving*. Den Haag: Sdu.

Duyvendak, J.W. (2004). *Een eensgezinde, vooruitstrevende natie. Over de mythe van 'de' individualisering en de toekomst van de sociologie*. Amsterdam: Vossius Pers (inaugural speech).

Duyvendak, J.W. and P. van der Graaf (2001). *Opzoomeren, stille kracht?* Utrecht: Verwey-Jonker Instituut.

Duyvendak, J.W. and M. Hurenkamp (eds.) (2004). *Kiezen voor de kudde. Lichte gemeenschappen en de nieuwe meerderheid.* Amsterdam: Van Gennep.

Duyvendak, J.W. and R. Rijkschroeff (2004). 'De bronnen van het integratiebeleid', *Sociologische Gids,* 51 (1) 3-17.

Duyvendak, J.W., R. Rijkschroeff and T. Pels (2005). *A multicultural paradise? The cultural factor in Dutch integration policy,* Paper presented at the ECPR Conference 2005, Budapest.

Duyvendak, J.W. and J. Uitermark (2005). 'De Opbouwwerker als Architect van de Publieke Sfeer'. *Beleid en Maatschappij,* 32 (2), 76-89.

Duyvendak, J.W. and T. Nederland (2006, in press) *New Frontiers for Identity Politics? Stretching and Limiting Identity in the Dutch Patients' Health Movement.* Utrecht: Verwey-Jonker Institute.

Dzur, A.W. (2004a). 'Civic Participation in Professional Domains: An Introduction to the Symposium'. *The Good Society,* 13 (1), 3-5.

Dzur, A.W. (2004b). 'Democratic Professionalism: Sharing Authority in Civic Life'. *The Good Society,* 13 (1), 6-14.

Eddy, D.M. (1990). 'Clinical Decision Making: From Theory to Practice. Designing a Practice Policy: Standards, Guidelines and Options'. *Journal of the American Medical Association, 22,* 3077-3084.

Eklund, L. (1999). *From Citizen Participation towards community Empowerment: An Analysis on Health Promotion from a Citizen Perspective.* Tampere: University of Tampere.

Engelen, E. (2005). 'De strijd om de instelling'. *Socialisme and Democratie,* 62 (5), 10-21.

Entzinger, H. (2003). 'The Rise and Fall of Multiculturalism: The Case of the Netherlands' In C. Joppke and E. Morawska, *Toward Assimilation and Citizenship: Immigrants in Liberal Nation-States.* New York: Palgrave.

Essen, van G., H. Meihuizen and F. Peters (2001). *Arbeid in zorg en welzijn. Integrerend OSA-rapport 2001.* Tilburg: Organization for Strategic Labour Market Research.

Etzioni, A. (ed.) (1969). *The Semi-Professions and their Organization: Teachers, Nurses Social Workers.* New York: The Free Press.

Exworthy, M. and Halford, S. (eds.) (1999). *Professionals and the New Managerialism in the Public Sector.* Buckingham: Open University Press.

Fagan, J. (2002). 'Policing Guns and Youth Violence'. *Future of Children,* 12 (2), 133-151.

Favell, A. (1998). *Philosophies of Integration: Immigration and the Idea of Citizenship in France and Britain.* Hampshire and New York: Palgrave McMillan.

Ferlie, E., L. Ashburner, L., Fitzgerald, A. Pettigrew (1996). *The New Public Management in Action.* Oxford: Oxford University Press.

Fermin, A.M.E. (1997). *Nederlandse politieke partijen over minderhedenbeleid 1977-1995.* Reeks Migrant en Stad 2. Amsterdam: Thesis Publishers

Fisher, C.M. (1998). *Resource Allocation in the Public Sector.* London: Routledge.

Fletcher, R.H., S.W. Fletcher and E.H. Wagner (1991). *Clinical Epidemiology. The Essentials.* Baltimore: Williams & Wilkins.

Flint J. (2002). 'Social Housing Agencies and the Governance of Anti-Social Behaviour'. *Housing Studies*, 17 (4), 619-637.

Foster, P. and P. Wilding (2000). 'Whither Welfare Professionalism?', *Social Policy & Administration* 34, 2, 143-59.

Foucault, M. (1978). *The History of Sexuality*. New York: Pantheon.

Frank, R. (2002). 'Integrating Homeopathy and Biomedicine: Medical Practice and Knowledge Production among German Homeopathic Physicians'. *Sociology of Health & Illness*, 24 (6), 796-819.

Frankford, D.M. (1997). 'The Normative Constitution of Professional Power'. *Journal of Health Politics, Policy and Law* 22, 1, 186-221.

Freeman, R. (2000). *The Politics of Health in Europe*. Manchester: Manchester University Press.

Freidson, E. (1970). *Professional Dominance: The Social Structure of Medical Care*. New York: Atherton.

Freidson, E. (1972). *Profession of Medicine*. New York: Dodd, Mead & Co.

Freidson, E. (1986). *Professional Powers: A Study of the Institutionalizations of Formal Knowledge*. Chicago: The University of Chicago Press.

Freidson, E. (2001). *Professionalism: The Third Logic*. Cambridge: Polity Press.

Frijhoff, W. and M. Spies (1999). *1650. Bevochten eendracht*. The Hague: Sdu.

Fulford, K. (2003). 'Value-Based Mental Health'. In WHO (ed.), *Report of the Sixth Meeting of the European National Counterparts for the WHO Mental Health Programme*. Madrid: WHO.

Gallagher, J. (2003). 'Specialties in Transition: The Case of Oral and Maxillofacial surgery' in C. Davies, (ed.) *The Future Health Workforce*. Basingstoke: Macmillan.

Gambrill, E. (2005). 'Critical Thinking, Evidence-Based Practice and Mental Health'. In S. Kirk (ed.) *Mental Disorders in the Social Environment: Critical Perspectives*. New York: Columbia University Press, pp. 247-269.

Gareau, F.H. (1986). 'The Third World Revolt against First World Science: An Explication Suggested by the Revolutionary Pedagogy of Paulo Freire'. *International Journal of Comparative Sociology* 27 (3-4), 172-189.

Gastelaars, M. (1985). *Een geregeld leven. Sociologie en sociale politiek in Nederland 1925-1968*. Amsterdam: SUA.

Gastelaars, M. (1997). *Human Service in Veelvoud. Een typologie van dienstverlenende organisaties*. Utrecht: SWP Publishers.

Gastelaars, M. and J. Vermeulen (2000). 'On Location. Cultural Pluralism and the Organizational Relevance of the "Here" and "Now"'. In M. Gastelaars (ed.) *On Location: The Relevance of the 'Here' and 'Now' in Organizations*. Maastricht: Shaker, pp. 9-26.

Geddes, J. and P. Harrison (1997). 'Closing the Gap between Theory and Practice'. *British Journal of Psychiatry*, 171, 220-225.

Gemeente Rotterdam (2003). *Kadernotitie sociale Integratie in de moderne Rotterdamse samenleving*. Rotterdam: Gemeente Rotterdam.

Gerhard, U., T. Knijn and J. Lewis (2002). 'Contractualization'. In B. Hobson, J. Lewis and B. Siim (eds). *Contested Concepts in Gender and Social Politics*. Cheltenham: Edward Elgar, pp. 105-140.

Gezondheidsraad (2000). *Van Implementeren naar Leren. Het Belang van Tweerichtingsverkeer tussen Praktijk en Wetenschap in de Gezondheidszorg*. Den Haag: Gezondheidsraad.

Giddens, A. (1991). *Modernity and Self-Identity.* Cambridge: Blackwell.

Giddens, A. (1998). *The Third Way: The Renewal of Social Democracy.* Cambridge: Polity Press.

Gilbert, N. (2002). *The Transformation of the Welfare State.* Oxford: Oxford University Press.

Goewie, R. (1986). *Dienstverlening aan culturele minderheden. Evaluatie van samenwerkingsprojecten vanuit het algemeen maatschappelijk werk.* 's Gravenhage: NIMAWO.

Gradener, J. (2003). Zinloze zelfkritiek. *Tijdschrift voor de Sociale Sector,* 57 (5), 5-10.

Grit, K. and P.L. Meurs (2005). *Verschuivende verantwoordelijkheden: dilemma's van zorgbestuurders.* Assen: Koninklijke Van Gorcum.

Gruyter, R. de (2004). 'Persoonsgebonden budget: geen garantie op goed gebruik'. *Tijdschrift voor de Sociale Sector,* 58 (1/2), 4-7.

Guadagnoli, E. and P. Ward (1998). 'Patient Participation in Decision-Making'. *Social Science and Medicine,* 47 (3), 329-339.

Gunaratnam, Y. and G. Lewis (2001). 'Racialising Emotional Labour and Emotionalising Racialised Labour: Anger, Fear and Shame in Social Welfare'. *Journal of Social Work Practice* 15, 2, 131-148.

Haan, I. de and J.W. Duyvendak (2002). *In het hart van de verzorgingsstaat: het ministerie van Maatschappelijk Werk en zijn opvolgers (CRM, WVC, VWS) 1952-2002.* Zutphen: Walburg Pers.

Haar, M. van der and M. Gastelaars (2004). 'Between essentialisms and everyday negotiations: Social work practice in a culturally plural society'. Paper presented at the International Conference Multiculturalisation: An International Perspective on the Ideology of Multiculturalism and the Practice of Multiculturalisation, Utrecht.

Hafferty, F.W. and D.W. Light (1995). 'Professional Dynamics and the Changing Nature of Medical Work'. *Journal of Health and Social Behavior,* Extra Issue 1995, 132-153.

Hafferty, F.W. and J.B. McKinlay (eds.) (1993). *The Changing Medical Profession: An International Perspective.* New York and Oxford: Oxford University Press.

Haines, A. and A. Donald (1996). *Getting Research Findings into Practice.* London: BMJ.

Hajer, R. (1981). *Volwassenenvorming – beleid en democratisering.* Amersfoort: NCVO.

Hall, C., S. Sarangi and S. Slembrouck (1997). 'Moral Construction in Social Work Discourse'. In Britt-Louise Gunnarsson, Per Linell and Bengt Nordberg (eds.) *The Construction of Professional Discourse.* London: Longman, pp. 265-291.

Hall, C., S. Sarangi and S. Slembrouck (1999). 'The Legitimation of the Client and the Profession: Identities and Roles in Social Work Discourse'. In S. Sarangi and C. Roberts (eds) *Talk, Work and Institutional Order: Discourse in Medical, Mediation and Management Settings.* Berlin: Mouton de Gruyter, pp. 293-322.

Harris, D. (2003). *Profiles in Injustice.* New York, The Free Press.

Harrison, S. (1999). 'Clinical Autonomy and Health Policy: Past and Futures'. In M. Exworthy and S. Halford (eds.) *Professionals and the New Managerialism in the Public Sector.* Buckingham: Open University Press, pp. 50-64.

Harrison, S. and C. Pollitt (1994). *Controlling Health Professionals: The Future of Work and Organisation in the NHS,* Buckingham: Open University Press.

Harrison, S. and W.I.U. Ahmad (2000). 'Medical Autonomy and the UK State 1975 to 20025'. *Sociology* 34, 1, 129-146.

Harrison S. and C. Smith (2004). 'Trust and Moral Motivation: Redundant Resources in Health and Social Care?'. *Policy and Politics* 32, 3, 371-86

HCI (Haut Conseil á l'Intégration) (1991). *Pour un modèle français d'intégration: premier rapport annuel.* Paris: La Documentation Française.

Healy, K. and C. Peile (1995). 'From Silence to Activism: Approaches to Research and Practice with Young Mothers'. *Affilia* 10 (3), 280-298.

Hood, C. (1991). 'A Public Management for all Seasons?' *Public Administration,* 69 (1), 3-19.

Hueting, E. and R. Neij (1991). 'Sociale zorg in grootstedelijke gebieden in beleidsmatig perspectief', In P. den Hoed (ed.) *Maatschappelijk werk en de stad: vijf preadviezen.*'s-Gravenhage: WRR, pp. 169-220.

Hunter, D.J. (1997). *Desperately Seeking Solutions: Rationing Health Care.* London: Addison-Wesley Longman.

Hupe, P. and L. Meijs (2000). *Hybrid Governance.* The Hague: SCP.

Hutschemaekers, G. (2001). 'Onder professionals: hulpverleners en cliënten in de geestelijke gezondheidszorg'. *Maandblad Geestelijke Volksgezondheid,* 56, 806-831.

Hutschemaekers, G. (2002). *Onder professionals.* Nijmegen: SUN.

Hutschemaekers, G. (2003). 'Multidisciplinary Guidelines in Dutch Mental Health Care: Plans, Bottlenecks and Possible Solutions'. *International Journal of Integrated Care,* 3 (10), issn. 568-4156.

Hutschemaekers, G. and R. Smeets (2005). 'Multidisciplinaire richtlijnen in de GGZ. Stand van zaken en uitdagingen voor de toekomst'. In A.H. Schene, F. Boer, T.J. Heeren, J.P.C. Jaspers, B. Sabbe and J. van Weeghel (eds.) *Jaarboek voor psychiatrie en psychotherapie vol. 9.* Houten: Bohn Stafleu van Loghum, pp. 273-288.

Hutschemaekers, G. and C. van den Staak (in press). 'The Dutch Case: The Rise and Decline of a Separate Psychotherapeutic Profession in the Netherlands'. *International Journal of Psychotherapy.*

Hutschemaekers, G.J.M. and L. Neijmeijer (1998). *Beroepen in Beweging. Professionalisering en grenzen van een multidisciplinaire GGZ.* Houten: Bohn Stafleu Van Loghum.

Huysman, M. (2003). 'Communities of Practice: naar een tweede generatie kennismanagement'. In R. Bood and M. Coenders (eds.) *Communities of Practice: een innovatief perspectief op kenniswerken.* Deventer: Kluwer.

Idenburg, Ph. (1999). *Het gaat om mensen.* Amsterdam: Balans.

Illich, I.D. (1977). *Disabling Professions.* London: Boyars.

Imrie R. (2004). 'Governing the Cities and the Urban Renaissance'. In C. Johnstone and M. Whitehead (eds.) *New Horizons in British Urban Policy: Perspectives on New Labour's Urban Renaissance.* Aldershot: Ashgate, pp. 129-142.

Ireland, P. (2004). *Becoming Europe: Immigration, Integration, and the Welfare State.* Pittsburgh: University of Pittsburgh Press.

Irvine, D. (2003). *The Doctors' Tale: Professionalism and Public Trust.* Abingdon: Radcliffe Medical Press.

James, A. (1994). 'Reflections on the Politics of Quality'. In A. Connorand S. Black (eds.). *Performance Review and Quality in Social Care*. London: Jessica Kingsley.

Jervis, P. and S. Richards (1997). 'Public Management: Raising our Game'. *Public Money and Management*, 17 (2). 9-16.

Jobard, F. (2002). 'Compter les violences policières, faits bruts et mises en récit', *Questions pénales*, XV, 3, June.

Jobard, F. and M. Zimolag (2006). 'When policemen go to court. A study on outrage, rebellion and violence against policemen'. *Questions pénales*, XVIII, 2. March.

Johnson, T. (1995). 'Governmentality and the Institutionalization of Expertise', In T. Johnson, G. Larkinand M. Saks(eds.) *Health Professions and the State in Europe*. London: Routledge.

Johnsonn, M. (2003). *Street Justice: A History of Police Violence in New York City*. Boston: Beacon Press.

Joppke, C. (1996). 'Multiculturalism and immigration: a comparison of the United States, Germany, and Great Britain'. *Theory & Society*, 25 (4): 449-500.

Joppke, C. (2004). 'The Retreat of Multiculturalism in the Liberal State: Theory and Policy'. *The British Journal of Sociology*, 55(2): 237-257.

Jordan, B. (2000). *Social Work and the Third Way: Through Love as Social Policy*. London: Sage.

Kaasenbrood, A. (1995). *Consensus als criterium. De ontwikkeling, de verpreiding en het gebruik van richtlijnen voor goed psychiatrisch handelen*. Utrecht: NcGv.

Kaasenbrood, A., T. Kuipers and B. van den Werf (2004). *Dilemma's in de psychiatrische praktijk*. Houten: Bohn Stafleu Van Loghum.

Kampman, M., G. P. Keijsers, C.A.L. Hoogduin and G. J. Hendriks (2002). 'A Randomized, Double-Blind, Placebo-Controlled Study of the Effects of Adjunctive Paroxetine in Panic Disorder Patients Unsuccessfully Treated with Cognitive Behavioural Therapy Alone'. *Journal of Clinical Psychiatry*, 63 (9), 772-777.

Kanters, H., W. van der Windt and M. Ott (2004). *Geen wildgroei managers in de zorg*. Utrecht: Prismant.

Katznelson, I. (1981). *City Trenches*. New York: Pantheon.

Kaufman, H. (1980). *The Administrative Behavior of Federal Bureau Chiefs*. Washington: Brookings Institution.

Kjaer, A.M. (2004). *Governance*. Oxford: Polity Press.

Kmietovicz, Z. (2004). 'Consumer advocate says GMC changes still don't go far enough'. *British Medical Journal* 328, 1338, (5 June).

Knijn, T. (1999). 'Strijdende zorglogica's in de kinderopvang en de thuiszorg: marktprincipes in de sociale zorg'. In C. Brinkgreve and P. van Lieshout (eds) *Geregelde gevoelens. Collectieve arrangementen en de intieme leefwereld*, Maarssen: Elsevier/De Tijdstroom, pp. 93-110.

Knijn, T. (2000). 'Marketization and the Struggling Logics of (Home) Care in the Netherlands'. In M. Harrington Meyer (ed.) *Care Work: Gender, Class and the Welfare State*. New York and London: Routledge, pp. 232-248.

Klerman, G.L. (1990). 'The Psychiatric Patient's Right to Effective Treatment: Implications of Osheroff vs. Chestnut Lodge'. *American Journal of Psychiatry*, 147 (4), 409-418.

Koenis, S. (1993). *De precaire professionele identiteit van sociaal werkers*. Utrecht: NIZW.

Kohnstamm, J. (2004). *Een herkenbare staat: investeren in de overheid. Rapport van de werkgroep verzelfstandigde overheidsorganisaties*. Den Haag: Ministerie van Binnenlandse Zaken en Koninkrijkszaken.

Kooiman, J. and M. van Vliet (1993). 'Governance and public management'. In K.A. Eliassen and J. Kooiman (eds) *Managing Public Organisations: Lessons from Contemporary European Experiences*. London: Sage.

Koopmans, R. and P. Statham (2000). 'Migration and Ethnic Relations as a Field of Political Contention: An Opportunity Structure Approach' In R. Koopmans and Statham P. (eds.) *Challenging Immigration and Ethnic Relations Politics: Comparative European perspectives*. Oxford and New York: Oxford University Press, pp. 13-56.

Koopmans, R., P. Statham, M. Giugni and F. Passy. (2006). *Contested Citizenship: Political Contention over Migration and Ethnic Relations in Western Europe*. Minneapolis: University of Minnesota Press.

Kremer, M. and L. Verplanke (2003). *New Managerialism and the Left Hand of the State. Professionals, States and Citizens*. Paper presented at the first conference of the European Social Policy Association, Copenhagen, 13-15 November.

Kremer, M. and L. Verplanke (2004). *Opbouwwerkers als mondige professionals*. Den Haag: LCO.

Kremer, M. and L.Verplanke (forthcoming). *De mondige opbouwwerker?* (provisional title) The Hague: National Community Work Centre.

Kruithof, K. (2005). *Doctors' Orders*. Unpublished Doctoral Thesis, Rotterdam.

Kuypers, P. (1993). 'Kwaliteit en zorg'. In L. Raymakers (ed.) *Zorg voor pedagogische kwaliteit*. Assen: NVO.

Kwakman, K. (1999). *Leren van docenten tijdens de beroepsloopbaan. Studies naar professionaliteit op de werkplek in het voortgezet onderwijs*. Nijmegen.

Kwakman, K. (2003). *Anders leren, beter werken*. Nijmegen: Hogeschool van Arnhem en Nijmegen.

Laan, G. van der (2003). 'De professional als expert in practice-based evidence'. *Sociale Interventie*, 12 (4), 5-16.

Laat, M. de and R. Poell (2003). 'Collectief leren op de werkplek: spontane en gestuurde initiatieven bijeenbrengen'. In R. Bood and M. Coenders (eds.) *Communities of Practice: een innovatief perspectief op kenniswerken*. Deventer: Kluwer.

Langley, J. and H. Mintzberg (1995). 'Opening Up Decision Making: The View from the Black Stool'. *Organization Science*, 6 (3), 260-279.

Larner W. and W. Walters (2000). 'Privatisation, Governance and Identity: The United Kingdom and New Zealand compared'. *Policy and Politics*, 28 (3), 361-377.

Latour, B. (1994). 'Pramatogonies: A Mythical Account of How Humans and Non-Humans Swap Properties'. *American Behavioral Scientist*, 37, 791-808.

LeGrand, J. and W. Bartlett (1994). *Quasi-Market and Social Policy*. Houndmills: Mcmillan.

Lipsky, M. (1980). *Street-Level Bureaucracy: Dilemmas of the Individual in Public Services*. NewYork: Russell Sage Foundation.

Lock, G. (2005). 'Nederland, Narcissus' paradijs'. In P. van Os (ed.), *Nederland op scherp. Buitenlandse beschouwingen over een stuurloos land*. Amsterdam: Bert Bakker.

Loopmans M. (2003). '"Opsinjoren" in Antwerpen: een geavanceerde vorm van governance [Opsinjoren in Antwerp: an advanced form of governance]'. *Agora*, 19 (5), 17-20.

Loopmans, M., J. Uitermark and F. De Maesschalck (2003). 'Against all odds: poor people jumping scales and the development of an urban policy in Flanders, Belgium'. *Belgeo*, 2 (3), 243-258.

Loopmans, M., S. Luyten and C. Kesteloot (2006). Urban policies in Belgium: a puff-pastry with a bittersweet aftertaste? In Van den Berg, L., Braun, E. & J. Vandermeer (eds.) *National Policy Responses to Urban Challenges in Europe*, Aldershot: Ashgate (forthcoming).

LSR (2003). *Richtlijn voor de diagnostiek en behandeling van angststoornissen.* Utrecht: Landelijke Stuurgroep Multidisciplinaire Richtlijnen in de GGZ.

LSR (2005). *Richtlijn voor de diagnostiek en behandeling van depressieve stoornissen.* Utrecht: Landelijke Stuurgroep Multidisciplinaire Richtlijnen in de GGZ.

Luborsky, L., L. Diguer and D.A. Seligman (1999). 'The Researcher's Own Therapy Allegiances: A "Wild Card" in Comparisons of Treatment Efficacy'. *Clinical Psychology: Science and Practice*, 6, 95-106.

Lucassen, L. and A.J.F. Köbben (1992). *Het Partitiële Gelijk. Controverses over het onderwijs in eigen taal en cultuur en de rol daarbij van beleid en wetenschap.* Amsterdam and Lisse: Swets & Zeitlinger.

Maatschappelijk Ondernemers Groep (2002). *Aan beide zijden van de voordeur. Positie en functies van het Algemeen Maatschappelijk Werk*. Utrecht: MO Groep.

Marangos, A. and J. Plantenga (2005). 'Kinderopvang. Loyaliteit als sterkste kracht'. In M. Hurenkamp and M. Kremer (eds.) *Vrijheid verplicht. Over tevredenheid en de grenzen van de keuzevrijheid*. Amsterdam: Van Gennep, pp. 59-76.

March, J.G. and J.P. Olsen. (1989). *Rediscovering Institutions*. New York: Free Press.

Margalith, I. and A. Shapiro (1997). 'Anxiety and Patient Participation in Clinical Decision-Making: The Case of Patients with Ureteral Calcul'. *Social Science and Medicine*, 45 (3), 419-427.

Marsh, D. (ed.) (1998). *Comparing Policy Networks*. Buckingham: Open University Press.

Mayer M. (2003). 'The Onward Sweep of Social Capital: Causes and Consequences for Understanding Cities, Communities and Urban Movements'. *International Journal of Urban and Regional Research*, 27 (1), 110-132.

McDonald, R. and S. Harrison (2004). 'The Micropolitics of Clinical Guidelines: An Empirical Study'. *Policy & Politics* 32, 2, 223-39.

McKee, L. et al. (1999) 'Medical Managers: puppetmasters or puppets?' in A. Mark and S. Dopson (eds.) *Organisational Behaviour in Health Care: The Research Agenda*. Basingstoke: Macmillan.

Meurs, P.L. and T.E.D. van der Grinten (2005). *Besturingsvragen in de zorg*. The Hague: Academic Service.

Miles, A., J. R. Hampton and B. Hurwitz (eds.) (2000). *NICE, CHI and the NHS Reforms: Enabling Excellence or Imposing Control?* London: Aesculapius Medical Press.

Mintzberg, H. (1983). *Structure in Fives*. Englewood Cliffs: Prentice Hall.

Mintzberg, H. (2004). *Managers, not MBAs*. San Fransisco: Berrett Koehler.

Mol, A. (2004). 'Klant of zieke? Markttaak en de eigenheid van de gezondheids-zorg'. *Krisis, tijdschrift voor empirische filosofie*, 5 (3), 3-24.

Moran, M. (1999). *Governing the Health Care State – A Comparative Study of the United Kingdom, the United States and Germany*. Manchester: Manchester University Press.

Morris, L. (1994). *Dangerous Classes: The Underclass and Social Citizenship*. New York: Routledge.

Munk, M. (2002). *Historische reconstructie van het debat rond het persoonsgebonden budget*. Unpublished paper. NIZW.

Mykhalovskiy, E. and L. Weir (2004). 'The Problem of Evidence-Based Medicine: Directions for Social Sciences'. *Social Science & Medicine*, 59, 1059-1069.

Nederland, T., J.W. Duyvendak and M. Brugman (2003). *Belangenbehartiging door de patiënten- en cliëntenbeweging: de theorie*. Utrecht: Verwey-Jonker Instituut.

Nederland, T. and J.W. Duyvendak (2004). *Effectieve belangenbehartiging. De kunst van effectieve belangenbehartiging door de patiënten en cliëntenbeweging: de prak-tijk*. Utrecht: Verwey-Jonker Instituut.

Newman, J. (2001). *Modernising Governance: New Labour, Policy and Society*. London: Sage.

Newman, O. (1972). *Defensible Space: Crime Prevention through Urban Design*. New York: MacMillan.

NIVEL (Nederlands Instituut voor onderzoek van de gezondheidszorg) (2004). *Evaluatie versterking eerstelijns GGZ: een onderzoeksprogramma om het beleid ter versterking van de eerstelijns GGZ te evalueren: eindrapportage landelijk onder-zoek*. Utrecht: NIVEL.

Noordegraaf, M. (2000). *Attention! Work and Behavior of Public Managers amidst Ambiguity*. Delft: Eburon.

Noordegraaf, M. (2004). *Management in het publieke domein. Issues, instituties en instrumenten*. Bussum: Coutinho.

Noordegraaf, M. and P.L. Meurs (2002) Verwarde managers. Professionalisering van managers in de zorg, *M 56 (3)*, 22-39.

Noordegraaf, M. and T. Abma (2003). 'Management by Measurement?' *Public Administration*, 81(4), 853-871.

Nuis, J.D.L., C.W.M. Dessens, W.G. van Hassel and A.B. Hoogenboom (2004). *Particulier speurwerk verplicht*. Den Haag: Koninklijke Vermande (Forensische Studies, deel 13).

O'Malley P. and D. Palmer (1996). 'Post-Keynesian policing'. *Economy and Society*, 25 (2), 137-155.

O'Neill, O. (2002). *A Question of Trust, The BBC Reith Lectures*. Cambridge: Cambridge University Press.

Ocqueteau, F. (2002). 'La réforme française au miroir des polices de proximité étrangères'. *Les Cahiers de la sécurité intérieure*, 39, 173-183.

Oevermann, U. (2000). 'Mediziner in SS-Uniformen: Professionalisierungs-theoretische Deutung des Falles Münch'. In H. Kramer (ed.), *Die Gegenwart der NS-Vergangenheit*, Berlin and Vienna: Philo Verlagsgesellschaft, pp. 18-76.

Offringa, M., W.J.J. Assendelft and R.J.P.M. Scholten (2000). *Inleiding in evidence-based medicine. Klinisch handelen gebaseerd op bewijsmateriaal*. Houten: Bohn Stafleu van Loghum.

Osmond, J. and I. O'Connor (2004). 'Formalising the Unformalized: Practitioners' Communication of Knowledge in Practice'. *British Journal of Social Work* 34, 677-692.

Oudenampsen, D.G. (1999). *De patiënt als burger, de burger als patiënt*. Ph.D. dissertation, Utrecht Universiteit, Utrecht: Verwey-Jonker Instituut.

Parker, D. and R. Lawton (2000). 'Judging the Use of Clinical Protocols by Fellow Professionals'. *Social Science and Medicine*. 51, 5, 669-677.

Parsons, T. (1964). *The Social System*. New York: Free Press.

Parsons, T. (1968). 'Professions'. In David Sills (ed.) *International Encyclopedia of the Social Sciences*. New York: Macmillan, pp. 536-547.

Peile, C. and M. McCouat (1997). 'The Rise of Relativism: The Future of Theory and Knowledge Development in Social Work'. *British Journal of Social Work* 27, 343-360.

Perrow, C. (2002) [1984]). *Normal Accidents*. Princeton: Princeton University Press.

Peters, T. and N. Austin. (Fall, 1985). MBWA (Managing by Walking Around). *California Management Review*, 28 (1), 9-34.

Pfadenhauer, M. (2004). 'Professionelle Organisation als Lernkulturen am Beispiel ärztlicher Fortbildung'. In Sybille Adenauer (ed.) *Kompetenzentwicklung 2004. Lernförderliche Strukurbedingungen*. Münster: Waxman, pp. 255-297.

Pickstone, J.V. (2000). *Ways of Knowing: A New History of Science, Technology and Medicine*. Manchester: Manchester University Press.

Pierson, P. (1994). *Dismantling the Welfare State? Reagan, Thatcher and the Politics of Retrenchment*. Cambridge: Cambridge University Press.

Pincock, S. (2003). 'Patients Put their Relationship with their Doctors as Second Only to that with their Families'. *British Medical Journal* 327, 581 (13 September).

Plemper, E., I. Abdulwahid van Bommel, J. Avezaat and R. Ramsaran (eds) *Wankele waarden. Levenskwesties van moslims belicht voor professionals*. Utrecht: Forum, Instituut voor Multiculturele ontwikkeling.

Pols, J. (2004). *Good care. Enacting a complex ideal in long-term psychiatry*. Utrecht: Trimbos instituut.

Pollitt, C. (1993). *Managerialism and the Public Services*. Oxford: Blackwell.

Pollitt, C. (2003). *The Essential Public Manager*. Berkshire: Open University Press.

Pollitt, C. and G. Bouckaert (2000). *Public Management Reform*. Oxford: Oxford University Press.

Potter, J. and M. Wetherell (1987). *Discourse and Social Psychology: Beyond Attitudes and Behaviour*. London: Sage.

Power, M. (1994). *The Audit Explosion*. London: Demos.

Power, M. (1999). *The Audit Society*. Oxford: Oxford University Press.

Pressman, J. L. and A. Wildavsky. (1984), *Implementation*. Berkeley: University of California Press.

Prins, B. (2000 [2004]). *Voorbij de onschuld. Het debat over integratie in Nederland*. Amsterdam: Van Gennep.

Putnam, R. (2000). *Bowling Alone: The Collapse and Revival of American Community*. New York: Simon & Schuster.

Raad voor de Volksgezondheid en Zorg/RVZ (2003). *Van patiënt tot klant.* Zoetermeer: RVZ.

Radstaeke, L. (2005). *Mensen maken de Stad.* Part of student research project, Department of Sociology, University of Amsterdam.

Raelin, J.A. (1986). *The Clash of Cultures.* Boston: Harvard Business School Press.

Reed, M. (1996). 'Expert Power and Control in Late Modernity: An Empirical Review and Theoretical Synthesis'. *Organization Studies* 17, 4, 573-97.

Reich, R. (1991). *The Work of Nations.* New York: Knopf.

Rhodes, R.A.W. (1997). *Understanding Governance: Policy Networks, Governance, Reflexivity and Accountability.* Buckingham: Open University Press.

Rijkschroeff, R.A.L. (1989). *Ondersteuning van participatie in de geestelijke gezondheidszorg.* Ph.D. dissertation, Amsterdam: University of Amsterdam.

Rijkschroeff, R., J.W. Duyvendak and T. Pels (2004). *Bronnenonderzoek Integratiebeleid.* Den Haag: Sdu.

Ritzer, G. (1993). *The McDonaldization of Society: an Investigation into the Changing Character of Contemporary Social Life.* Thousand Oaks: Pine Forge Press

RMO (Raad voor Maatschappelijke Ontwikkeling) (2000). *Aansprekend burgerschap. De relatie tussen de organisatie van het publieke domein en de verantwoordelijkheid van burgers.* The Hague: Council for Social Development.

Rose N. (1996). 'The Death of the Social? Re-figuring the Territory of Government'. *Economy and Society,* 25 (3), 327-356.

Saake, I. (2004). 'Theorien der Empirie. Zur Spiegelbildlichkeit der Bourdieuschen Theorie der Praxis und der Luhmannschen Systemtheorie'. In G. Nollmann and A. Nassehi (ed.) *Bourdieu und Luhmann.* Frankfurt am Main: Suhrkamp, pp. 85-117.

Sackett, D.L., S.E. Strauss, W.S. Richardson, W. Rosenberg and R.B. Haynes (2000). *Evidence-Based Medicine: How to Practice and Teach EBM.* Edinburgh, London and New York: Churchill Livingstone.

Saint-Upéry, M. (1997). Préface to Mike Davis, *City of Quartz.* Paris: La Découverte, I-XII.

Salas, D. (2005). *La volonté de punir.* Paris: Hachette.

Sarangi, S. and C. Roberts (1999). 'The Dynamics of Interactional and Institutional Orders in Work-related Settings'. In S. Sarangi and C. Roberts (eds) *Talk, Work and Institutional Order: Discourse in Medical, Mediation and Management Settings.* Berlin: Mouton de Gruyter, pp. 1-57.

Sayles, L. (1989). Leadership, *Managing in Real Organizations.* New York: McGraw-Hill.

Scheffer, P. (2000). Het multiculturele drama. *NRC Handelsblad,* 29 Jan. 2000

Schnabel, P. (2000). *De Multiculturele Illusie.* Utrecht: Forum.

Schön, D. (1983). *The Reflective Practitioner. How Professionals Think in Action.* New York: Basic Books.

Scholte, M (2003). 'Het bewijs is (nog) niet geleverd'. *Tijdschrift voor de sociale sector,* 57 (10), 20-23.

Scholte, M. and G. Hutschemaekers (2004). 'Gooi de veranderingen van de afgelopen jaren niet op een hoop!' *Maatwerk* (4), 6-11.

Schweder, R.A. (1990). 'Cultural Psychology – What Is It?' In: *Cultural Psychology Essays on Comparative Human Development.* J.W. Stigler, R.A. Schweder and G.S. Herdt (eds.). Cambridge: Cambridge University Press, pp. 205-232.

Scott, J.C. (1998). *Seeing like a State.* New Haven: Yale University Press.

Scott, W.R. (1995). *Institutions and Organizations.* Thousand Oaks: Sage.

SCP (Sociaal en Cultureel Planbureau) (2002). *Sociaal en Cultureel Rapport. 2002 De kwaliteit van de quartaire sector.* The Hague: Social and Cultural Planning Bureau.

Sehon, S.R. and D.E. Stanley (2003). 'A Philosophical Analysis of the Evidence-Based Medicine Debate'. *BMC Health Services Research* (July 21), 3-14.

Selznick, Ph. (1984 [1957]). *Leadership in Administration: A Sociological Interpretation.* Berkeley: University of California Press.

Sennett, R. (1998). *The Corrosion of Character.* New York: Norton.

Sennett, R. (2003). *Respect in a World of Inequality.* New York and London: Norton and Company.

Sheaff, R., K. Smith and M. Dickson (2004). 'Is GP Restratification Beginning in England?'. *Social Policy and Administration* 36, 7, 765-779.

Shotter, J. and M. Billig (1998). 'A Bakhtinian Psychology: From Out of the Heads of Individuals and Into the Dialogues Between Them'. In M. Mayerfield Bell and M. Gardiner (eds.) *Bakhtin and the Human Sciences,* pp. 13-29. London: Sage Publications.

Smith, M.J. (1993). *Pressure, Power & Policy: State Autonomy and Policy Networks in Britain and the United States.* New York: Harvester Wheatsheaf.

Smith, S.R. and M. Lipsky (1994). *Nonprofits for Hire: The Welfare State in an Age of Contracting.* Cambridge: Harvard University Press.

SOMA vzw and OCMW Antwerpen (2000). *Sociaal Impulsfonds Antwerpen: evaluatierapport programma 1997-1999 [Social Impulse Fund Antwerp: Evaluation Report 1997-1999].* Antwerpen: Stad Antwerpen.

Soysal, Y.N. (1994). *Limits of Citizenship: Migrants and Postnational Membership in Europe.* Chicago: University of Chicago Press.

Spierts, M., L. Veldboer, P. Vlaar and F. Peters (2003). 'De professionaliteit gesmoord'. *Tijdschrift voor de Sociale Sector* 57, 5, 10-15.

Stacey, M. (1992). *Regulating British Medicine.* Chichester: Wiley.

Stad Antwerpen (2002). *Feestkrant 5 jaar Opsinjoren [Celebration of 5 years of Opsinjoren].* Antwerpen: Dienst Samenlevingsopbouw.

Stad Antwerpen (2003). *De kracht van de stad: Beleidsplan Stedenfonds 2003-2007 [A City's Strength: City Fund Policy Plan 2003-2007].* Antwerpen: Stad Antwerpen.

Stad Antwerpen and OCMW Antwerpen (1997). *Beleidsplan Sociaal Impulsfonds 1997-1999 [Policy Plan Social Impulse Fund 1997-1999].* Antwerpen: Stad Antwerpen.

Stad Antwerpen and OCMW Antwerpen (2000). *Beleidsplan Sociaal Impulsfonds 2000-2002 [Policy Plan Social Impulse Fund 2000-2002].* Antwerpen: Stad Antwerpen.

Stehr, N. (1994). *Knowledge Societies.* London: Sage Publications.

Sternberg, R.J. and J.A. Horvarth (eds.) (1999). *Tacit Knowledge in Professional Practice.* Mahwah: Lawrence Erlbaum.

Stichweh, R. (1996). 'Professionen in einer funktional differenzierten Gesellschaft'. In A. Combe and W. Helsper (ed.) *Pädagogische Professionalität. Untersuchungen zum Typus pädagogischen Handelns.* Frankfurt/Main: Suhrkamp, pp. 49-69.

Sting (2004). *Ervaringen van PGB zorgverleners met het PGB.* Sting: Utrecht.

Stone, A.A. (1990). 'Law, Science, and Psychiatric malpractice: A Response to Klerman's Indictment of Psychoanalytic Psychiatry'. *American Journal of Psychiatry*, 147 (4), 419-427.

Stout, C. and Hayes, R. (eds.) (2005). *The Evidence-Based Practice: Methods, Models, and Tools for Mental Health Professionals*. Hoboken: Jon Wiley & Sons.

Strauss, A.L., S. Fagerhaugh, B. Suczek and C. Wiener (1997). *Social Organisation of Medical Work*. New Brunswick London: Transaction Publishers.

Strauss, S.E., W.S. Richardson, W. Rosenberg and R.B. Haynes (2005). *Evidence-Based Medicine: How to Practice and Teach EBM*. 3rd edition. Edinburgh, London and New York: Churchill Livingstone.

Struijs, A. and F. Brinkman (1996). *Botsende waarden. Ethische en etnische kwesties in de hulpverlening*. Utrecht: NIZW.

Strull, W.M., B. Lo and Ch. Gerald (1984). 'Do Patients Want to Participate in Medical Decision Making?' *Journal of American Medical Association (JAMA)*, 252 (21), 2990-2994.

Stüssgen, R. (1997). *De nieuwe patiënt op weg naar autonomie*. Ph.D. dissertation, Interdisciplinary Social Science Department, Utrecht University.

Sullivan, W. (2004). 'Can Professionalism Still Be a Viable Ethic?' *The Good Society*, 13 (1), 15-20.

SWA (Stichting Wijkalliantie) (2004). *Wijkalliantie. Verzet een wereld in de wijk*. Amsterdam: Stichting de Wijk.

Swaan, A. de (1982), *De mens is de mens een zorg. Opstellen 1971-1981*. Amsterdam: Meulenhoff.

Swaan, A. de, C. Brinkgreve and J. Onland (1979). *De Opkomst van het Psychotherapeutisch Bedrijf*. Utrecht and Antwerpen: het Spectrum.

Tanenbaum, S.J. (2005). 'Evidence-Based practice as Mental Health Policy: Three Controversies'. *Health Affairs*, 24 (1), 163-174.

Terry, L.D. (1996). *Leadership of Public Bureaucracies*. Thousand Oaks: Sage.

Thorne, M.L. (2002). 'Colonizing the New World of NHS Management: The Shifting Power of Professionals'. *Health Services Management Research*, 15, 1, 14-26.

Timmerans, S. and E.S. Kolker (2004). 'Evidence based medicine and the reconfiguration of medical knowledge'. *Journal of Health and Social Behavior*, 45 (Supplement), 177-193.

Tonkens, E. (1996). 'Voor gek gehouden, voor gek gezet. Constructivisme en maakbaarheid in de anti-psychiatrie'. *Krisis. Tijdschrift voor Filosofie*, 16 (1), 29-39.

Tonkens, E. (1999). *Het zelfontplooiingsregime. De actualiteit van Dennendal en de jaren zestig*. Ph.D dissertation, KUN / Amsterdam: Bert Bakker.

Tonkens, E. (2002). 'De mondige burger op de markt van welzijn en geluk'. In R. P. Hortulanus and J.E.M. Machielse (eds) *Modern burgerschap, Het sociaal debat*. The Hague: Elsevier, pp.83-94.

Tonkens, E. (2003). *Mondige burgers, getemde professionals. Marktwerking, vraag sturing en professionaliteit in de publieke sector*. Utrecht: NIZW (Netherlands Institute for Care and Welfare).

Trappenburg, M. (2005). *Gezondheidszorg en democratie*. Inaugural address, EUR.

Trappenburg, M. and M. de Groot (2001). 'Controlling Medical Specialists in the Netherlands. Delegating the Dirty Work. In M.A.P. Bovens, P. 't Hart and B.

Guy Peters (eds.) *Success and Failure in Public Governance*. Cheltenham/ Northampton: Edward Elgar, pp. 219-237.

Trouw (2005). 'Jeugdhulp boos over vervolging voogd; zaak Savanna', 12 March 2005.

Tshui, M.S. and C.H. Cheung (2004). 'Gone with the Wind: The Impact of Managerialism on Human Services'. *British Journal of Social Work* 34, 437-442.

Tuchman, B. (1980). *De waanzinnige veertiende eeuw*. The Hague: Elsevier.

Tucker, D.J. (1996). 'Eclecticism Is Not a Free Good: Barriers to Knowledge Development in Social Work. *Social Services Review* (Sept.), 401-434.

Uitermark, J. (2003). 'De sociale controle van achterstandswijken [The Social Control of Deprived Neighbourhoods]'. *Nederlandse Geografische Studies, 322*, Utrecht and Amsterdam: Koninklijk Nederlands Aardrijkskundig Genootschap.

Uitermark, J. (2005). *Anti-Multiculturalism and the Governance of Ethnic Diversity*, Paper presented at the Annual Meeting of the American Association of Geographers, 5-9 April 2005.

Uitermark, J. and J.W. Duyvendak (2004). *De weg naar sociale insluiting. Over segregatie, spreiding en sociaal kapitaal*. The Hague: RMO.

Uitermark, J. and J.W. Duyvendak (2005a). *Civilizing the City: Revanchist Urbanism in Rotterdam (the Netherlands)*. Working paper Amsterdam School for Social Science Research, University of Amsterdam.

Uitermark, J. and J.W. Duyvendak (2005b). *Participatory logic in a mediated age. Neighbourhood governance in the Netherlands after the multicultural drama*. Paper presented at the Cities as Social Fabric: Fragmentation and Integration Conference, Paris, 30 June-2 July, 2005.

Uitermark, J., U. Rossi and H. van Houtum (2005). 'Reinventing Multiculturalism: Urban Citizenship and the Negotiation of Ethnic Diversity in Amsterdam', *International Journal Urban and Regional Research*, 29(3): 622-640.

Ungar, M. (2004). 'Surviving as a Social Worker: Two Ps and three Rs of Direct Practice'. *Social Work*, 488-496.

Verhaak, C.M., F.W. Kraaimaat, A.C.J. Staps and W.A.J. van Daal (2000). 'Informed Consent in Palliative Radiotherapy: Participation of Patients and Proxies in Treatment Decisions', *Patient Education and Counseling*, 41, 63-71.

Verkaar, E. (1991). *Strategisch gedrag van kategorale patiëntenorganisaties*. Ph.D. dissertation, EUR / Utrecht: NIZW.

Vigoda, E. (2002). 'From Responsiveness to Collaboration: Governance, Citizens and the Next Generation of Public Administration'. *Public Administration Review*, 62 (5), 527-540.

Vogd, W. (2002). 'Professionalisierungsschub oder Auflösung ärztlicher Autonomie. Die Bedeutung von Evidence Based Medicine und der neuen funktionalen Eliten in der Medizin aus system- und interaktionstheoretischer Perspektive'. *Zeitschrift für Soziologie*, 31 (4), 294-315.

Vogd, W. (2004a). 'Ärztliche Entscheidungsfindung im Krankenhaus bei komplexer Fallproblematik im Spannungsfeld von Patienteninteressen und administrativ-organisatorischen Bedingungen'. *Zeitschrift für Soziologie*, 33 (1), 26-47.

REVIEW COPY

Policy, People, and the New Professional

De-professionalisation and Re-professionalisation in Care and Welfare

Edited by Jan Willem Duyvendak, Trudie Knijn, and Monique Kremer

Published by Amsterdam University Press
Distributed by the University of Chicago Press

Domestic Publication Date: February 15, 2007

192 p.   Paper • $47.50   ISBN 978-90-5356-885-9

For more information, please contact Harriett Green by phone at (773)702-4217, by fax at (773)702-9756, or by e-mail at hg@press.uchicago.edu.

Please send two copies of your published review to:

Publicity Director, THE UNIVERSITY OF CHICAGO PRESS
1427 E. 60th Street, Chicago, Illinois 60637, U.S.A. Telephone 773-702-7740

ORDERING INFORMATION

Orders from the U.S.A. and Canada:

The University of Chicago Press
Order Department
11030 South Langley Avenue
Chicago, Illinois 60628
U.S.A.
Telephone: 1-800-621-2736 (U.S.A. only);
(773) 568-1550
Facsimile: 1-800-621-8476 (U.S.A. only);
(773) 660-2235
Pubnet @ 202-5280
WWW: http://www.press.uchicago.edu

Orders from the United Kingdom and Europe:

The University of Chicago Press
c/o John Wiley & Sons Ltd.
Distribution Centre
1 Oldlands Way
Bognor Regis, West Sussex PO22 9SA
UNITED KINGDOM
Telephone: (0) 1243 779777
Facsimile: (0) 1243 820250
Internet: cs-books@wiley.co.uk
WWW:
http://www.wiley.com/WorldWide/Europe.html

Orders from Japan:

Booksellers' orders should be
placed with our agent:
United Publishers' Services, Ltd.
Kenkyu-sha Building
9, Kanda Surugadai 2-chome
Chiyoda-ku, Tokyo
JAPAN
Telephone: (03) 3291-4541
Facsimile: (03) 3293-3484
Libraries and individuals should place their
orders with local booksellers.

Orders from Australia, New Zealand, South Pacific, Africa, the Middle East, China (P.R.C.), Southeast Asia, India, Mexico, Central and South America:

The University of Chicago Press
International Sales Manager
1427 E. 60th Street
Chicago, Illinois 60637
U.S.A.
Telephone: (773) 702-7740
Facsimile: (773) 702-9756
Internet: dblobaum@press.uchicago.edu

Orders from Korea, Hong Kong, and Taiwan, R.O.C.:

The American University Press Group
3-21-18-206 Higashi Shinagawa
Shinagawa-ku, Tokyo, 140
JAPAN
Telephone: (03) 3450-2857
Facsimile: (03) 3472-9706
Internet: andishg@po.iijnet.or.jp

Vogd, W. (2004b). *Ärztliche Entscheidungsprozesse des Krankenhauses im Spannungsfeld von System- und Zweckrationalität: Eine qualitativ rekonstruktive Studie*. Berlin: VWF.

Vogd, W. (2005). *Systemtheorie und rekonstruktive Sozialforschung – Versuch einer Brücke*, Leverkusen: Verlag Barbara Budrich.

Vos, R., R. Houtepen and K. Horstman (2003). 'Evidence-Based Medicine and Power Shifts in Health Care Systems'. *Health Care Analysis*, 10 (3), 319-328.

Vries, S. de (2000). *Psychosociale hulpverlening en vluchtelingen*. Utrecht: Pharos.

Vuijsje, H. (1997). *Weldenkend Nederland sinds de jaren zestig*. Amsterdam: Contact.

Vulto, M. and M. Morée (1996). *Thuisverzorging als professie. Een combinatie van hand, hoofd en hart*. Utrecht: De Tijdstroom.

VWS (Ministerie van Volksgezondheid, Welzijn en Sport) (2004). *Brancherapport Welzijn en Sport: 2000-2003*. Den Haag: VWS.

Waaldijk, B. (1999). 'Marie Kamphuis en de wijde wereld van het maatschappelijk werk'. In B. Waaldijk, J. van der Stel and G. van der Laan (eds.) *Honderd jaar sociale arbeid. Portretten en praktijken uit de geschiedenis van het maatschappelijk werk*. Assen: Van Gorcum, pp. 113-127.

Waaldijk, B., J. van der Stel and G. van der Laan (eds.) (1999). *Honderd jaar sociale arbeid. Portretten en praktijken uit de geschiedenis van het maatschappelijk werk*. Assen: Van Gorcum.

Watts, R.D., D.M. Griffith, J. Abdull-Adil (1999). Sociopolitical Development as an Antidote for Oppression-Theory and Action. *American Journal of Community Psychology* 27 (2). 255-271.

Weick, K. (1995). *Sensemaking in Organizations*. Newbury Park: Sage.

Wenger, E. (1998). *Communities of Practice: Learning, Meaning and Identity*. Cambridge and New York: Cambridge University Press.

Wenger, E., R. McDermott and W. Snyder (2002). *Cultivating Communities of Practice: A Guide to Managing Knowledge*. Boston: Harvard Business School Press.

West, L. (2004). 'Doctors on the Edge: A Cultural Psychology of Learning and Health'. In P. Chamberlayne, J. Bornatand U. Apitzsch (eds.), *Biographical Methods and Professional Practice*. Bristol: The Policy Press.

Whitehead, M. (2004). 'The Urban Neighbourhood and the Moral Geographies of British Urban Policy'. In C. Johnstone and M. Whitehead (eds.) *New Horizons in British Urban Policy: Perspectives on New Labour's Urban Renaissance*. Aldershot: Ashgate, pp. 59-73.

Wieviorka, M. (1992). *La France raciste*. Paris: Le Seuil.

Wikan, U. (2002). *Generous Betrayal: Politics of Culture in the New Europe*. Chicago and London: University of Chicago Press.

Wilde, R., de (1992). *Discipline en Legende: De identiteit van de sociologie in Duitsland en de Verenigde Staten 1870–1930*. Amsterdam: Van Gennep.

Wilensky, H.L. (1964). 'The Professionalization of Everyone?' *American Journal of Sociology*, 70 (2), 137-158.

Wilson, J.Q. (1989). *Bureaucracy: What Government Agencies Do and Why They Do It*. New York: Basic Books.

Wilson, J.Q. and G. Kelling (1982). 'The Police and Neighborhood Safety: Broken Windows'. *Atlantic Monthly*, 249 (3), 29-38.

Woolhandler, S., T. Campbell and D.U. Himmelstein (2003). 'Costs of Health Care Administration in the United States and Canada'. *The New England Journal of Medicine*, 349 (8), 768-775.

WRR (Wetenschappelijke Raad voor het Regeringsbeleid) (2000). *Het borgen van het publieke belang* (Rapport aan de regering nr. 56). The Hague: Sdu.

WRR (Wetenschappelijke Raad voor het Regeringsbeleid) (2003). *Waarden, normen en de last van het gedrag* (Rapport aan de regering nr. 68). Amsterdam: Amsterdam University Press.

WRR (Wetenschappelijke Raad voor het Regeringsbeleid) (2004). *Bewijzen van goede dienstverlening* (Rapport aan de regering nr. 70). Amsterdam: Amsterdam University Press.

Yeatman, A. (1994). *Postmodern Revisioning of the Political*. New York and London: Routledge.

Yperen, T. van (2003). 'Verhoging van de effectiviteit in de jeugdzorg'. In *Nederlands tijdschrift voor Jeugdzorg* 6, 290-301.

Zauberman, R. and R. Levy (2003). 'The French State, the Police and Minorities'. *Criminology*, 41 (4), 1065-1100.

Zwart, F. de (2005). 'The Dilemma of Recognition: Administrative Categories and Cultural Diversity'. *Theory and Society*, 34, 137-169.

Index